Peace with Pain

Peace with Pain

Your Guide to Life in a Malfunctioning Body

by Jenna Sundell

Electric Bliss Publishing

Quote from Rama used with permission from
the Frederick P. Lenz Foundation for American Buddhism.
How to Make Friends with God lecture,
© Frederick P. Lenz Foundation for American Buddhism;
To listen to these and other talks by Dr. Lenz (Rama) please see the extensive Resource Library on the Rama Meditation Society site (ramameditationsociety.org).

Quote from Shankara used with permission from
Vedanta Press, Hollywood CA.
Shankara's Crest Jewel of Discrimination: Timeless Teachings on Nonduality translated by Swami Prabhavananda and Christopher Isherwood. © 1947, 1975 Vedanta Society of Southern California.

Quote from Ramakrishna used with permission from
the Ramakrishna-Vivekananda Center.
The Gospel of Sri Ramakrishna, translated into English with an Introduction by Swami Nikhilananda.
© 1942 by Swami Nikhilananda, New York,
Ramakrishna-Vivekananda Center.

Dancing Girl icons made by Freepik from www.flaticon.com. Flaticon is used under a Creative Commons Attribution 3.0 United States License.

Cover and Interior design by Phillip Tommey
www.philliptommeydesign.com

ISBN-13: 978-0692305935
(Electric Bliss Publishing)
ISBN-10: 0692305939

This book is dedicated to all who suffer
from the effects of chronic pain:
patients, their loved ones, and
their health care providers.
May the challenges you face cause you to grow
into higher and more beautiful states of mind.

Acknowledgements

This book began over 12 years ago, and there have been more people than I can count who have helped bring it into being, so please excuse my inability to mention everyone by name. I owe my deepest gratitude to my husband, Jim. With his infinite patience and love, Jim has supported me in all of my work and is the grounding force in my life. Thank you to my friend and partner at Dharma Center, Lynne Miller, who has traveled with me on the journey of offering meditation classes to the public, and who braved readings of the early and very painful versions of this book. The depth of her compassion knows no bounds. I also must thank all of my health care professionals – even the ignorant ones who caused me more pain – because they gave me the inspiration to start this book for the benefit of others with chronic pain. To my current body workers and doctors, thank you for doing what you do, as it allows me to do all that I do. All of the students, teachers, supporters, and volunteers of Dharma Center have shown me people really do want to be happy in this crazy world, and it is you who inspired me to finish this project. My thanks go to Maggie Susman (www.maggiesusman.com) for creating the beautiful artwork in the Short Instructions. For those of you who took on the extra work of proofreading, and especially my tough task master editor, Rosleen Reynolds, you have my gratitude for improving this book. Thank you all for helping to birth this book. If I met you at any point, in person or not, then you probably aided me in the completion of this work. With my deepest gratitude: THANK YOU!

May any suffering I experience – past, present, or future – be transmuted into Joy and Peace for the benefit of all sentient beings.

Table of Contents

Author's Note 1

Short Instructions 6
   Meditation 7
   Mindfulness 8

The Nature Of Pain 10

My Experiences, My Labels 15

The Pitfalls Of Pity 25

The Power Of Responsibility. 30

Journal Writing:
  Exploring The Gory Details 36

Meditation Practice 58
   What Is Meditation? 59
   Benefits Of Daily
     Meditation Practice 60
   Preliminary Meditation Practices 61
   How To Meditate. 64
   Using Pain During Meditation 72
   Inner Light 76
   A Space Of Your Own 79
   Meditation Tools 83
   Selecting A Meditation Class 88
   Meditation Tips 92
   Playing With Opposites 94
   Intentional Contemplation 98
   Meditation Recap 104

The Mind 106
   What Is Mindfulness? 110
   Mindfulness Practice:
     Making Everyday Life A Meditation. 113
   Smile Before Sleeping 116
   Using Karma To Your Advantage 118
   Fleeting Feelings Of Emotions 124
   Don't Take Anything Personally 127
   Dealing With Other People 131
   A Little Secret About Stress 141

Personal Happiness &
   Recreating Your Self Image 145
Impeccability 151
Goals And Having
   A Purpose For Being 156

Taking Care Of The Body 161
   Pacing 162
   Body Rhythms:
      Time To Eat, Time To Sleep 169
   Decisions About
      Disability Income 176
   Budget Basics 185
   Treatments And Therapies
      (A Limited List) 201
      Nutrition 205
      Body Work 210
      Medication 227
   Building Your Health Care Team 236

Terminal Sentence 241

Mystery Of The Month 245
   Chronic Fatigue Syndrome (CFS) 248
   Fibromyalgia (FM) 250
   Chronic Myofascial Pain (CMP) 252
   Temporomandibular Joint Dysfunction (TMD) 254
   Lyme Disease and Co-infections 258

Tips For Pain Flares 261

Tips For Daily Living 266

Taking Refuge 271

The Most Important Moment 274

Making Peace With Pain 276

Deeper Still 279

Resources 280
   Books 280
   Musical Artists For Meditation 285
   Movies 286
   Websites 289

About The Author 294

Please remember: it is very important for you to work with your health care provider as you experiment with different treatments and lifestyle changes. I am not a doctor and I have no medical training. Nothing in this book should be construed as medical, legal, or financial advice. Proceed at your own risk, as practicing these techniques may cause excessive happiness.

Author's Note

This book began as an answer to two questions asked by a psychologist running the pain management class I attended. A group of us, all facing a life of chronic pain, sat together, hoping to find a better way to live. At the beginning of class, the psychologist asked: "What makes you a survivor?" and "What is enough?"

When I got home, I tried to answer those questions by writing in my journal. Soon I realized simply surviving was not enough for me. I wanted to thrive, be happy, and do activities I loved. Over time I learned I could live a bright, happy, and productive life – just not in the way I used to.

I spent the first few years of my illness clinging to my old self. I pushed myself to walk three blocks every day to the cliffs overlooking the ocean while dreaming of hiking miles and miles in the mountains. In front of my computer, I tortured myself by updating my resume and creating an impressive portfolio of my work as a computer consultant. A large binder grew each month with samples of programming code, project plans, reports I had designed, and user guides I had written. Every time I looked at my resume, I felt crushed by the knowledge I would not be able to hold a job even if I could find someone to hire me. Once my portfolio was complete, I put it in the closet with all of my business clothes.

One day after meditating, I finally took an honest look at myself. I saw a sick, disabled woman. I had tried to beat my body into submission, but in the end the body won the war. I could barely walk a block without stopping to rest, it took only ten minutes at the computer before I could no longer type, I randomly fell on the floor, and the doctors told me all they could do was treat the pain with drugs. I felt like giving up, and some days I did. My boyfriend could do nothing but watch and try to stay out of the line of fire as I fought my body.

As I spun through the darkness of self-pity, my training as a Buddhist monk kept pulling me to a calm, almost surreal space. My ego pushed reason after reason why I should be miserable, yet something deeper and stronger within me laughed. I cried, I whined to my boyfriend, I got angry at myself and the world, occasionally I would smile – and through it all, a tiny warrior part of me kept slowly plugging along, a half-step at a time.

Without even realizing it, I had been creating a new life for myself. It wasn't until I let go of the jet-setting computer consultant I once was that I saw I did indeed have a good life.

During the early stages of my illness in 1998, my friend and I opened Dharma Center, where I taught meditation classes. Dharma Center was our way of honoring the memory of our teacher, Rama, and giving back some of what he had given us. Sitting with eager new students provided me the opportunity to revisit all of the basics of my practice. And for an hour each week, I forgot about my body's health issues. The pain was still there; it just wasn't as important as sharing the teachings with these new students.

Other Rama students learned that I had written a book about the study, and begged me for copies. In September 2001, I published *Worlds of Power, Worlds of Light* for them. Physically unable to promote the book, I was thrilled when it began selling purely by word of mouth advertising. Suddenly, I realized I was an author and a meditation teacher.

Teaching meditation challenged me to keep growing even when I wanted to crawl in a hole and cry. As I met thousands of people, all with unique challenges, I saw in action the most basic lesson Rama taught: Every experience is an opportunity to practice the Path.

Through my classes, I met a special population of students who were also struggling with chronic pain. They would often show up alone, and then stay after class to ask specific questions relating to the practice and pain. They are the ones who inspired me to complete this book, not only for them, but also for the ones who cannot attend a meditation class like the ones I teach.

Because of this Path, I do not live in ordinary human consciousness. If I did, I would be trapped in bed moaning in pain. Over years of practice, I have learned to perceive reality from a different vantage point.

This learning process goes on forever. Every moment has the potential to degrade into a battle against the ego, with its self-importance, its precious personal history, and its non-stop self-pity. The ego, while a necessary component of the body in this world, is transient. Boundless, infinite Eternity is the real master, with the ego merely facilitating the interactions of the physical world. A perfect healthy body, although beneficial, is not required for spiritual growth. The work of training the ego is challenging; the rewards of ecstasy are beyond rational explanation. To see firsthand the immensity of Eternity opens the door to unfathomable bliss. To know Eternity and consciously stand embracing the mystery is freedom.

The pain and illness that invaded my body forced me to let go of who I thought I was or should be. Throughout the struggles I faced many different selves and tried to cling to each of them. During my transformations I discovered none of those faces were mine. I am no longer the person crippled by pain, nor am I the woman who triumphed over pain. I am no longer any particular person. Every day I am something entirely new.

Spiritual practice is the guiding force of my life. I rely upon it to bring forth the strength necessary to thrive in a fulfilling, beautiful life even though my body does not always cooperate. I humbly offer you these teachings, which have given me the power to know unconditional joy and peace in the midst of pain and sorrow.

Every moment we are presented with opportunities to explore the mystery and wonder of Eternity. All that is required for growth is a willingness to open the mind and heart to the infinite possibilities waiting within you.

~Jenna Sundell
9/21/14

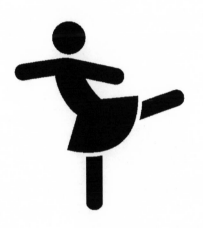

Short Instructions

"You may not be able to alter your condition in life,
but you can love."
~Rama

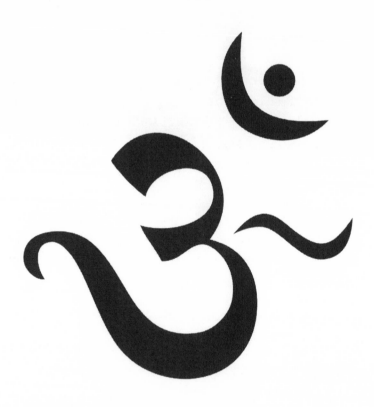

Meditation

➤ Sit up comfortably. Use pillows to help keep your back straight if necessary.

➤ Focus on the symbol in this section. It is the Sanskrit symbol for Aum, sometimes spelled OM. (It's pronounced *Aauummm*.)

➤ Focus all of your attention on the picture; look at every detail in the image. Ignore any thoughts or feelings that arise by pulling your attention back to the picture. You may need to re-focus many times; each time you re-focus your attention, you are making your mind stronger.

➤ Either out loud or silently in your mind, say Aum several times as you continue to focus on the picture. Over and over, pronounce: Aauummm, Aauummm, Aauummm, Aauummm...

➤ Just for a few moments, try it NOW!

➤ Beginning today, give yourself at least one minute each day to practice by returning to this page.

Mindfulness

When you're not seated in meditation, practice mindfulness. Mindfulness means to be fully present in the moment. To do this, you first must learn to control your mind. Here are three simple steps to gain control. It's not always easy; however, it is simple and very effective.

1. Pay attention to the thoughts and feelings within your mind. Ask, "What am I thinking? What am I feeling?" Give the mind state you are in a label.

2. Ask yourself if this mind state is beneficial. Is it a fun place to be? Do you want to continue living in this mind state?

3. If it's not bright and happy, change it. You change your thoughts by consciously placing your attention on something else. Each time you catch an unpleasant thought in your mind, focus on beauty or gratitude. Look around and use whatever you see that is beautiful, or whatever you can feel grateful for at this moment. It could be a color, a tree, a nice pair of shoes, the sun reflecting on a piece of glass, or being thankful you have a place to live, or that you can breathe, etc. Keep focusing on the beautiful object or the feeling of gratitude until your mind shifts into a more beautiful and peaceful state. Your ego will

give you a list of reasons to keep your attention on the thoughts creating misery; put your ego and reasoning aside for now. Continue bringing your focus back to beauty and/or gratitude for as long as it takes to shift to a higher and happier state of mind. Once you've shifted, relax in the beauty and gratitude of this present moment.

Please Note: Your body may be screaming in pain, but your mind doesn't have to join it. (I know that's a hard habit to break.) Make the body as comfortable as possible, and then move your mind into beauty and gratitude. You will feel happier, but don't take my word for it; try it now.

The Nature Of Pain

At 3:00am
This dream called pain
Wakes me in the night
While even the cat dozes
At the end of the bed
Piercing my inner ear and jaw
And stinging the top of my head
As if an anvil has fallen
From the sky

Pain sucks. In all its myriad forms, pain still sucks. Pain has hundreds of different qualities and expressions; it still sucks. There's the beaten by baseball bats type of pain; there's burning, stabbing, throbbing, crushing pain; there's head-splitting and pin-prick pain; there's pain that feels like you're walking on nails; there's the pain that makes you feel like you're wading through molasses; and of course, we cannot forget the deep aching pain. No matter how you slice it, pain sucks.

Overall, there are two types of pain: physical pain and mental pain. Or, as the lawyers like to put it: pain and suffering. So, from now on, when I refer to suffering, I mean the anguish of your mind. And when I refer to pain, I mean the physical type – the kind that makes your body say *Ouch*.

Pain is the body's messenger to tell the brain that

something is not right. It is a vital part of the human body's functioning. Without pain, we would scald ourselves in the shower when the water is too hot. Pain stops us from causing more damage when we step on a piece of broken glass, sprain our ankles, or when we try to pick up something too heavy for our muscles to bear. Pain, even though it can suck, is an important helper in our daily lives.

For some of us though, pain is a tyrant. It is always screaming, demanding attention. Like the Little Boy Who Cried Wolf, it can be difficult to tell when the pain actually needs medical care. When the doctors and other health care providers have done all they can to diagnose the cause and relieve the pain, we have to learn to live with the tyrant. We have to learn its patterns, qualities, and changes in intensity. Then we have to vigilantly watch for any new faces of pain that reveal themselves, so we know if the body needs any new types of treatment.

With a tyrant always yelling at you, it's natural to suffer. *Will the pain ever stop? What if I have something else wrong and I can't tell because the pain is always so intense? Why me?* Just a few of the questions your ego will ask, over and over, and over again. Unfortunately, those questions usually don't have answers.

One thing I have learned after more than a dozen years of constant pain and many more years of hard-core Buddhist practice is this:

> *Pain is a physical sensation that can be ignored.*
> *Suffering is a mental state that can be changed.*

Pain is a physical sensation. The senses are very

interesting, and through them we explore hundreds of different experiences every moment. Pain has a high priority in the mind's programming because it is crucial to our physical survival. However, it is only one of thousands of possible sensations.

When our attention is focused on pain, our awareness literally shrinks and the pain becomes our entire world. Once corrected, the pain recedes and our attention drifts to other sensations. Take a moment to explore some of the sensations you're experiencing right now: pain if you have it, the texture of your clothes against your skin, the softness of your cat's fur, the sound of birds chirping, the tap-tap of a neighbor hammering his porch, the scent of your friend's perfume, the sight of a tree swaying in the breeze, the temperature in the room, the coolness of your glass of water...all these things are happening right now, and there is even more beyond the senses.

When you are suffering, it is difficult to experience the more pleasant sensations. It's like watching a horror movie: you really don't want to see the blood and gore, yet you cannot pull your eyes off the screen. And even when the movie is over, the disturbing images may still haunt you. However, you do have the power to change the channel and watch something else.

Laughter is one way to deflect the intensity of pain and change your focus. Our response to pain is conditioned in us from when we are young. I learned this from my nephew when he was learning to walk. Each time he fell down, he would first quickly look around the room at the people. If someone smiled, he would giggle, push himself back up and start walking again. If someone instead gave him a pouty look and showed him pity, he would immediately start crying and not move until someone picked him up. In my own experiences with pain, I've found it much easier to move my attention to a higher state if I laugh when I feel the sensation of pain. Of course the first few times I saw my chiropractor, he thought I was a little weird, but he got over it when I told him the other option was screaming.

It's not easy to alter the focus of your mind when the pain is intense, however, it can be done. It's not easy living in suffering with a tyrant pounding your back all day long either. So for me, the choice to work hard at the practice of meditation and mindfulness is clearly a better alternative than living in misery. It's a choice I make every moment.

> *You are not your body.*
> *You are not your thoughts.*
> *You are not your emotions.*
> *You are not your feelings of intuition.*
> *You are not your dreams.*
> *You are not your mind.*
> *You are not your ego.*
> *You are none of these fragile things.*
> *You are merely having experiences in this physical*
> *reality that will not last.*
> *You are nameless – vast, eternal, love, light are words*
> *that can only allude to*
> *Your true nature.*

Take Action!

- ❖ Take a deep breath and notice the different sensations you feel right now.

- ❖ Notice the unpleasant sensations without recoiling away from them.

- ❖ Now move your attention to the pleasant sensations and let yourself enjoy them.

My Experiences, My Labels

One day, as I sat watching reruns on television, trying to ignore the pain racing around my body, I knew I needed to force myself eat something for lunch. My face and jaw hurt too much too chew, so I grabbed a high calorie, high fat nutrition drink from the refrigerator. With only 110 pounds on a 5'7" frame, I couldn't afford to lose any more weight. Within five minutes of finishing my liquid meal in a can, I felt a sharp spasm just below my ribcage. The next thing I knew, I was on the floor screaming.

By this time in my experience, pain was familiar to me. Every night I tossed and turned, working my muscles until I drifted off for 20 minutes, and then I would wake up sore and begin tossing and turning again. Every morning it felt like walking on nails as each muscle revolted from being asked to carry its own weight. For over three years, I had lived each and every moment with some part of my body complaining. This time however, the pain was new and more intense than anything I had ever experienced.

I dragged myself to the bathroom, where I vomited my liquid lunch. The pain continued to increase as more shrieks escaped my mouth. I crawled across the floor and managed to pull the phone from the coffee table, but I couldn't dial. Overwhelmed with this new twisting sensation of pain, my mind and fingers simply wouldn't work. I laid there fighting the screams as tears streamed down my face, knowing I needed help but at the same time knowing I couldn't function enough to dial and talk.

Suddenly the phone rang. I pushed the button and squeaked out: "help." Lynne, my friend and partner at Dharma Center, was on the other end. She rushed over and called 911 and Jim, my then boyfriend, now husband.

As we waited for the ambulance, Lynne held my hand. She looked at me and said, "Focus on Rama, focus on your teacher." Once the words left her lips, I remembered my practice. A profound shift occurred and my mind became completely clear. The pain remained just as intense. I still couldn't sit up. Yet I was completely calm and coherent. I knew on every level of my being I am not this fragile body. I knew that this experience of pain was transient and I was not the pain I was feeling.

The EMT's arrived and put an oxygen mask on my face as we drove to the hospital. With the oxygen, the pain began to quiet. It felt surreal to have such intense pain of an unknown cause and be completely at peace at the same time. I remember feeling joy and gratitude when I looked at Jim because he had made it home from work in time to ride to the hospital with me.

Of course, my calm demeanor completely confused the emergency room doctor. I tried to explain the severity of the pain, but without the uncontrollable screams and tears, he just didn't get it. After an x-ray and some blood tests, he diagnosed me with constipation. In accordance with the policy of most emergency rooms, I was "treated and streeted" – a shot of morphine for the pain and a shot of milk of magnesia for the constipation, and then sent home.

The next day I saw my primary care doctor, who didn't want to contradict the ER doctor. He recommended more laxatives and a day or two of fasting. A few days later, the pain continued, and although it was not as intense, there was definitely something new and very wrong in my belly.

I phoned the doctor, and he wanted me to wait two weeks to see a specialist. Realizing he did not understand the severity of the pain, I called upon my inner New York bitch – the project manager within me who knew how to get things done. With the same ruthless determination I had learned in Manhattan's corporate boardrooms, I told the secretary: "No, I will not wait two weeks. I'm still in pain and I need the doctor to order whatever test will show us what's wrong today." I used calm and forceful pressure to get my point across, being careful not to slip into anger. I had already learned angry patients are easy to ignore.

Twenty minutes later, she called back with an appointment for an abdominal ultrasound the next morning. The ultrasound revealed a gallbladder bursting with gallstones, and I was scheduled for surgery right away.

This extreme example of how I live with pain is just that, one example. I share it with you not to convince you of anything, but rather to show you what I have learned. Your experience will undoubtedly be different. Even knowing that, we still have the irresistible urge to compare experiences and labels. We want to know we are not alone, and we want to determine how much effort to put into trying what has worked for another. I have no doubt you will find your own way to peace in the midst of pain, just as I have found mine.

My gallstone attack and resulting sudden Satori – that instant realization of being more than a fragile body – occurred in a moment, yet it came about because of years of daily practice. Before this dramatic example, I had experienced the transcendence of pain on many occasions; however it was always subtle and easy to forget.

My adventure with chronic pain, that 24/7, every moment of every day pain, slowly crept up on me when I was 27, right in the middle of my fantastic and successful life as a Buddhist monk, computer consultant, writer, and happy homemaker. Doctors labeled my body issues with a long list of names like TMJ Dysfunction, Fibromyalgia, Chronic Fatigue Syndrome, Chronic Myofascial Pain, Endometriosis, chronic ovarian cysts, Interstitial Cystitis, and most recently, Lyme disease with co-infections like Babesia and Bartonella.

After the doctors found the gallstones spilling out of my gallbladder, I celebrated the victory over vomiting, even though it took two years and a trip to the ER to find the cause. In a happy coincidence, the gallbladder surgery also fixed the Irritable Bowel Syndrome, but not before I learned where the bathroom is in every store in every neighborhood I've ever visited.

Years later, antibiotic treatment for Toxoplasmosis and the "late-stage" Lyme disease cured me of my stomach acid and GERD. Again I celebrated – one less pill, whoo-hoo! The antibiotics also stopped the drunken loopy-ness that made me fall down at random moments (yea!); apparently my alcohol-free drunken moments were caused by the Toxoplasmosis. However, even after a full year of antibiotic treatment, the pain persists within my body. One doctor tells me the Lyme disease and co-infections will take stronger and longer doses of antibiotics; while another doctor tells me it's not Lyme disease because my blood tests came back indeterminate. All I know for certain is the constant pain and fatigue limit my activity and force me under the label "disabled" and onto the couch for frequent rest breaks.

I've eaten mountains of pills, gone on strict diet regimens, and seen every type of MD, DO, DC, PT, and alternative care practitioner known in America. I've consulted Tibetan doctors, Chinese medicine specialists, and those skilled in Ayurveda. I've worn mouth splints to relax my jaw and used special pain relieving creams and massage tools and heating packs in all sizes, shapes and scents. A selection of ice packs dominates a section of my freezer, and I always have lavender bubble bath on hand to soothe my hundred-plus trigger points.

Before beginning one experimental treatment, my massage therapist created a map of my very own, personal trigger points. The theory was that over time, the trigger points would dissolve and the process could be documented by my body worker.

The treatment didn't work, but the map did improve my ability to communicate with doctors. When they ask where it hurts, I show them the picture of all the little X's, so when I say "It hurts everywhere" they know I am not exaggerating and I really do mean everywhere. They can see for themselves the extent of the trigger points. Apparently a picture really is worth a thousand words!

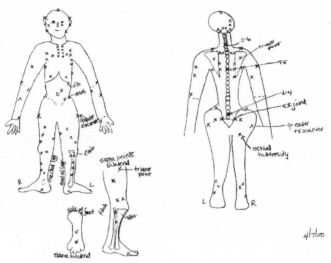

X = Trigger point, a knot in the muscle that often refers pain into adjacent muscles

Throughout the years, I've tried countless traditional and not so traditional things to fix my body. One friend even dragged me to a psychic healer who could only tell me he saw toxins in my body, but couldn't tell me where they were from or offer a solution to remove them. This, of course, prompted yet another batch of experiments designed to purify the cells of my body. Herbs and special diets dominated my consciousness, but I still did not find my remedy.

With every suggestion of a possible cure, or even a modicum of relief, I willingly boarded the roller coaster of hope and despair those of us with pain know all too well. We eagerly hear about the details as the cart goes click-click-click up the hill. We begin the treatment as we whoosh down the hill, filled with excitement and fear. Then the first corner nearly takes us out...the treatment doesn't seem to be doing anything, and maybe it's making things worse. But, wait, maybe I feel a little stronger, a little more energetic – we go up another hill, filling with hope. We rush down and around again and again, as the despair sets in and we realize the treatment didn't work the way we expected and we are suddenly back to where we started.

Even though I know that ride well, I still get tempted to hop on for a spin. I do it because there have been things that help some, and a little bit of relief is often worth the risk. Now that I'm older and have more experience, I look carefully before jumping on. I research the opportunity thoroughly and I check to see what else is going on in my life before I decide to begin the next experiment.

I've learned I need to choose my projects with discretion, whether they are body, writing, or teaching related. We never know exactly how the body will react to anything we put it through, and sometimes we wind up worse off than before. So I've learned to explore my options slowly, with eyes wide open.

As I've moved through all of these experiences, what has astonished me is the power of the labels we give to our experiences and to ourselves. These labels are descriptions we use to ground ourselves in an experience. They can help us, or they can keep us stuck in a rut. While my insurance company and doctors classify me as "disabled" it's a label I tend to use sparingly because it makes me feel heavy and burdened. The same is true of the names of the diseases I have been told I have. I understand the use and necessity of these labels in certain situations, but I also realize the power they have to weigh me down. When dealing with doctors, I remind myself that I am not my diagnosis.

Other labels have the power to lift me up, so I rely upon those often, especially when I experiment with treatments. My favorite label, the one I hold in my mind most often is Buddhist monk. My spiritual practice is my saving grace. At the end of the day, even when I get completely spun out from whatever particular roller coaster I find myself riding, I remember why I'm here in this body.

In the light of spiritual growth, a malfunctioning body doesn't matter so much, and can even be a blessing. As I've often said to my students, it is only when we decide we have suffered enough, that we finally devote ourselves fully to the spiritual path.

Shortly after being ordained, many fellow students started grumbling about the difficulty of the Path. Rama told us, "You can leave any time, but the door will follow you." The door he spoke of was the door of awareness we opened when we chose to become Buddhist monks. That awareness is now part of us, and no matter what we do, it will always be there. I am fortunate to have had already made the choice to follow the spiritual path before my body became ill. My experiences have been a brutal proving ground for the teachings, and whatever doubts I had in the past have been completely erased.

My days begin and end with meditation, and I strive to be present and mindful of all the moments in between. This body, with all of its complaints, is one of my greatest teachers. It forces me into the present with its screaming pain. The fatigue makes me sit when I want to run away. This body has taught me respect, kindness, and patience. Even though I still whine on occasion, for all of that, I am grateful.

Probably the toughest thing to explain is the realization my body and I can have very different experiences at the same time. Yes, the body is in severe pain. No, I'm not bummed out about it; I'm actually feeling the ecstasy of this moment. Yes, I would like my body to work normally. Yes, I miss hiking for ten miles in the mountains and practicing Aikido and the feel of my muscles working. Now in my muscles, I just feel the burning and aching and the random stabbing, not to mention how they don't always cooperate when I have plans for them. But that's not enough to destroy my peace of mind because I know with every fiber of my being I am not this fragile body.

This body is my vehicle, and I am responsible for taking care of it to the best of my ability. This vehicle, which allows me to have experiences in this crazy, wonderful, human world of all possible mind states, is precious. And even with its disability, this precious body is able to take me where I need to go to grow and share the light of Enlightenment in this world. And through this body, I experience constant severe pain, extreme ecstasy and profound peace, all at the same time each and every day. And I know the same is possible for you.

Take Action!

- ❖ What have your experiences with pain taught you?

- ❖ Labels can elevate us, or they can weigh us down. What labels do you have for yourself that elevate you?

- ❖ Make a list of these helpful labels; write one on each day of your calendar for the next week as a reminder to let your labels support you.

The Pitfalls Of Pity

Sit: silence within
Let stillness rule all actions
Love and Light, your guides

It is a socially accepted practice to pity those who are in pain. Pity is an expected reaction; those who do not show pity are called cold-hearted. Pity however, leads to many problems, especially for the person to whom the pity is directed. These problems include low self-esteem, a distorted self-image, loss of personal power, envy, and the lure to manipulate others. In a situation where the pain is temporary and short-lived, people shake off pity in a variety of ways and then go back to their normal, healthy lives. For people with chronic pain, pity can be a road leading to hell.

Many people in the world experience empathy, where they can actually feel the suffering of another as if it were their own. Obviously this is very uncomfortable. As a means of self-protection, a person transforms the empathy into sympathy or pity. In essence, the person separates herself from the person who is in pain. This person now can stand above the one in pain, saying "Oh you poor thing." Energetically, the impression is one of "I am better than you because you are helpless" pushing the person in pain further down. Sometimes whole groups of people get together to feel sorry for someone, where they unconsciously focus a great deal of energy that sends the message "you are helpless" to the person in pain. When confronted with this day after day for years on end, it is no wonder the person in pain begins to believe it.

Most people are well intentioned and do not mean to cause those of us who live in chronic pain any harm. They are simply following social protocol. That is unlikely to change in the near future, so we are put to the challenge of weeding out the damaging subtle messages we receive from others.

They actually believe they are helping by feeling sympathy for you; it shows they care about you. A remedy for this situation is to give the person a constructive way to help you. Even a small task you give them will allow them to express their concern for you. If there's nothing you need done, then telling them you are glad they are there is enough. Recognizing and fulfilling their desire to be of service turns their pity into a beneficial encounter for both of you.

Probably the biggest issue surrounding pity is the fact that people who feel deeply sympathetic will often go out of their way to help you. This is both a good and a bad thing. Sometimes we do need help, and it is important we ask for that help. Sometimes we just want something and we use pity to get it. Only you know where that line is, and it may change from day to day. One day I can get myself a glass of water; other days the short walk to the kitchen wipes me out for the rest of the evening. Using pity to manipulate others is a fast track towards a pit of despair. Unfortunately, many people don't see it until they are already in the pit, feeling like they can do nothing for themselves.

The good news: there is always a way out. You may not like your options, but there are always options. The first step is to take an honest inventory of your capabilities. *What can you do for yourself without increasing your pain? What can you do for yourself without causing a long-term increase in pain? How long will the pain last if you do it for yourself?* Once you have this information, you can weigh the benefits of doing the task for yourself versus asking someone else to do it for you. Sometimes I have to carry my water glass with two hands and it hurts, but I feel better about myself as a whole if I do it myself. For me, it's worth the short increase in pain. If I'm in a severe flare and have trouble standing up, I swallow my pride and ask for help.

It would be easy not to do the self-monitoring and let others do everything for me; however, this approach creates problems. The sympathetic message, "you are helpless" would be constantly reinforced by the action of letting people do everything for me. Over time, I may even begin to expect this special attention and forget to thank those that help. The people helping me may begin to feel resentful and taken advantage of, and then have to face the guilt for having those feelings. For me, that cycle is more difficult to live with than the constant self-monitoring and questioning, *Can I honestly do this for myself right now or not?*

This question is not a judgment on self-worth. It is simply a clinical assessment of the capabilities of the body. Basing your actions on an honest assessment will go a long way towards building respect for your body and your self as a whole.

At every moment, you have control of only the focus of your own mind. You cannot change or control another unless they let you. So when you experience pity from a friend or stranger, watch your mind carefully. How do you feel? Reinforce the idea that you are a valuable human being. Your intrinsic worth is exactly the same as everything else in existence, no more and no less. Remember the things you can do for yourself and allow yourself to do them. Communicate clearly with the people you spend time with when you need to rest, and follow through. If you say you need to rest, then find the first available place to sit until you feel better. Be prepared to let your companions go on without you if they are impatient. Feel good about taking care of your body as you rest. From this mind state of acceptance and honesty, compassion is born.

Compassion is entirely different than sympathy. Many people use the words interchangeably; however there is a dramatic difference from my point of view. One Buddhist teacher I met defined compassion as the sincere wish for others not to suffer. I define compassion as the act of seeing a person's true nature. To have compassion for another (or oneself) is the ability to look past the ego, past the body, past all the ideas of how you think someone is, and see him or her as an expression of Eternity, of God. In essence, you are Light, infinite and eternal. At the core of your being, beyond the ideas and ego-experiences, you are whole and complete. To recognize this in yourself and others is true compassion.

Compassion is the most wonderful gift you can give. By perceiving someone in this way, you provide a mirror that allows your friend to step out of his or her limited viewpoint and become something more. True compassion is rare in this world. It requires the empathetic person to move past the self-protection of sympathy, and accept the pain they see and feel as only one layer of experience. For compassion to emerge, you cannot fight the pain and sorrow. Instead you look deeply into its core and see the universal Light from which we all are formed.

 ## Take Action!

❖ Take an honest inventory of your capabilities. Where do you need assistance? What tasks are you able to do by yourself?

❖ Practice compassion right now by seeing yourself as an expression of Eternity, of God. Say to yourself: "I am an expression of Eternity. I am whole and complete."

❖ Whenever you experience self-pity or pity from others, practice compassion for yourself and them.

The Power Of Responsibility

Healing.
Releasing.
Flowing.
Explosions of pain within muscle and joint…
The space of meditation is available
At all times, in any place.

The Path I have begun to share with you is demanding. It involves taking full personal responsibility and an enormous amount of hard work, and it will cause you to change in ways I cannot even begin to describe. What awaits you is unconditional joy, laughter, fun, and profound peace of mind. The tyrant of pain will probably still be there, but playing a new role as a grumpy old friend who may want your attention but doesn't always get it. I can only point the way on this Path; it is you, my friend, who must walk it.

Don't believe anything you read in here – instead, allow yourself the time to experiment and see if it works for you. There are lots of options and approaches and even a few tricks, so if something doesn't work, try something else. What didn't work today may help you on a different day, so file it away for later.

One thing I must demand of you is complete and total honesty with yourself. You can lie to the rest of the world if you really want to, but always be honest with yourself. You are the only one who knows if you are being diligent with your practice or if you're slacking off. If you find yourself slipping into misery, an honest assessment of the state of your mind will reveal the way out. Or as a friend of mine once said: *Recognition is Liberation*.

The first step on this Path is taking full personal responsibility for the state of mind in which you are currently living, right now. This step does not involve creating any blame or guilt, or even asking why your mind is in that state. Simple acceptance of the fact that you are _____ (fill in the blank: depressed, sad, happy, angry, silly, bored, jealous – whatever it may be) and knowing you are indulging in that particular mind state now is enough. Don't concern yourself over how you usually feel; instead take a look at where your mind is right now, at this moment.

Of course you have a thousand and one reasons for being in that mind state. None of them matter. Not one little bit. Nope. Sorry. It doesn't matter if your best friend yelled at you five minutes ago for something you didn't do and that made you angry. The cold hard truth is you allowed yourself to hang onto the anger after it arose in your mind and you chose, consciously or not, to keep hanging onto it. So now you've probably moved your anger to me. Well, I don't care. I refuse to take it personally – I know better than to give someone else that kind of power over me.

That's what taking personal responsibility is really about; it's about taking back your personal power. No one can make you feel happy or sad or angry or anything else. Events can trigger these mind states, but it is always your choice whether or not to stay there, indulging in them. Unfortunately most people are never taught this, so they live their lives being pushed from one mind state to another by circumstance. While we can exert a little bit of influence over the physical world, we really cannot control it. Sometimes we cannot even control our own bodies. The only place we do have control is over the focus of our own mind.

So take an honest look at your mind state. Is it a fun, happy place? Or is it a scary, dark place? Call it what it is, without apologies, without excuses. Simply state it as a fact, and accept the truth of it.

Once you've done this, you may feel a little different. There may be a surge of emotion or a feeling of release. Or you may feel the mind state even more intensely. Let yourself feel whatever it is that you're feeling. Pretend for a moment you are a scientist and your mind is one of your experiments. Remember: You are not your mind state. You are not your house, either. But you do live in your house and in your mind state.

Now accept responsibility for being in that mind state. Don't turn it into a guilt trip or a self-pity party; those are just other states of mind. Say to yourself: "I accept responsibility for being in this mind state." Again, no excuses or apologies or reasons are needed. Simply accepting where you are and knowing you got yourself there is enough.

These two simple acts may be enough to give you the power you need to move almost automatically into a whole different state of mind, hopefully one that is much more fun. Essentially what you have done is found where your mind is on the map of possible experiences and put yourself in the driver's seat of the Mind's car. Only then can you drive yourself to a better place.

Although, I suppose you could hang out in that dark mind state and wait for the fairy godmother to bonk you on the head with her wand and then you'll be happy...until midnight anyway. But if you hate to wait, taking personal responsibility may be a better option.

There are many things that affect your state of mind, and sometimes mind states are symptoms of an illness. For example, if you've been depressed for more than two weeks in a row and there is no trigger for it, you could have a medical condition causing it. If you skip eating all day, you may feel aggravated. Or, if you start taking a new medication and find yourself filled with thoughts of worry, the anxiety could be a side effect of the drug. Another example is if you have chronic pain and you push yourself into exhaustion, you will most likely experience mind states of irritability and frustration. In this case, you can use the techniques in this book to pull yourself out of those mind states temporarily, but you will snap back over and over until you deal with the root cause.

Personal responsibility also means to take care of your body to the best of your ability. You get this body once, so why not take care of it as best you can? It's not the doctor's job to make you well. The doctor certainly has a great deal of information to help you figure out what your body needs for optimum functioning, but it's up to you to do it. You are the only one who can tell the doctor all of your symptoms and which ones are bothering you the most. You are also the only one who can judge whether or not the treatment is helping. Sometimes a medication may appear to be fixing the problem, but it's really only disguising the original problem and creating more problems for you. The doctor won't know this unless you report it. And you cannot report it if you are not aware of it. Begin now by paying attention to your mind, take responsibility for what you feed your mind and where you let your mind rest.

Now that you have taken the first difficult step of personal responsibility, you are ready to start working on your daily practice. Meditation will provide you with clean, pure energy as you strengthen your willpower. Then we will tackle mindfulness, an active form of meditation in which you learn to dance with the ego while interacting with the world. Through the twin practices you will discover the mysteries within you, waiting.

As you take this journey into awareness, please know this is a *practice*. You will make the same mistake over and over – there is only one mistake to make: the Buddha called it Attachment. That is the one and only cause of your suffering; it is what keeps you unaware of your true nature. Whenever you find yourself off balance in a dark mind state, look deep enough and you will find whatever you are attached to. The practice will teach you how to gain control over your mind and release the attachments keeping you stuck in the endless cycles of suffering. As you free yourself from the layers of attachment, you'll move closer to knowing your true nature: pure, perfect Light. Instead of suffering through life, you'll discover the play of existence, and see firsthand there's always more to experience. And just so you know, once you get out of the dark lower mind states, things get a whole lot more fun – no matter what is going on with the body.

Take Action!

❖   Stop for a moment and become aware of your state of mind.

❖   Give it a label, and notice what that state of mind feels like.

❖   Observe how the world looks to you from this state of mind.

❖   How does this state of mind affect your body?

Journal Writing:
Exploring The Gory Details

Journal writing provides a release like no other. On the blank page, you can express yourself without judgment and without censorship. By placing your thoughts and feelings on paper, you create distance from them. Writing for only yourself allows you to gain a clear view of where you are at that particular moment. When you see the words on the page, you can objectively decide how many of these ideas you want to continue to carry with you. During a single writing session, you can watch as you let go of the parts of yourself you no longer need and grow into the next brighter, stronger version of You.

The words you put on paper don't need to make sense to anyone else. Your journal is a private place for you to express whatever is floating around in the corners of your mind. One moment you may write about your pain and suffering, and the next your words may turn towards the silly fun experiences in your life. You may write about dreams or desires or fears. You may write about visiting with a friend or what you watched on television or your trip to the grocery store. Simply letting yourself write freely without editing, opens a door to exploring your mind.

Writing gives a voice to both the dark and the bright thoughts in your mind. When you put the thoughts that haunt you on paper, they lose the power they have over you. Instead of festering in the shadows of your mind, you bring them out into the light where they can dissipate. You can see them for what they are: just thoughts whirling around. Conversely, when you record your dreams and joys, you can consciously focus on them. Putting your beautiful thoughts and experiences on paper allows you to save the power of those moments.

Growth can be difficult to see because it happens moment by moment. If you have long hair, you may not notice for many months how much it has grown. The same is true with personal growth. Your journal will allow you to see how far you have come during the course of a year or two or three.

On the following pages, I have included some of my personal journal entries. They are snapshots of my experiences as I learned to deal with my illness. I hope these rambling words of pain, life, and light inspire you to begin your own private journal.

4/11/98

The road to recovery is a long one.
Day-by-day, I carry on, fighting
the pain. It drains me as I watch
from deep within,
a beam of light sustains me.

5/6/98

Knives pierce my shoulder on all sides, sending burning pain up my neck into my jaw. Yes, my shoulder is messed up. It hurts to lean back on it, but I lean anyway. I am frustrated and in pain no matter what I do. Doctors, massage therapists, and chiropractors – I'm sick of them all, but ignoring this pain is not working.

My throat is tight and I want to cry, but my tears have all dried up. In my mind, I resolve to push through the pain and be productive. My body refuses to cooperate. So I suffer.

There are better options to focus on: The sun feels good on my head. The wind chimes sing a joyous song with the morning birds.

I'm so tired of fighting. Will this war ever end?

I'm learning things about pain I never wanted to know.

When will I be strong enough to be who I am?

I am...a writer, a teacher, a systems analyst, a software tester, a lover, an artist, a biker, a Buddhist monk.

How am I being untrue to myself?

I pretend I can deal with the physical pain and become frustrated when I cannot. And this makes me feel weak, so I put up a front of false strength to protect myself. The facade keeps cracking. I want to write stories but I let the rest of my life get in the way.

Time is slipping between my fingers and I cannot catch it. I feel trapped within a nightmare, and I wake up only to find myself in yet another nightmare.

Jim makes me smile long enough to turn my mind to joyful thoughts. The pain of my body rips me to shreds and he is not able to hold me together. I fall like rain and collect myself in a puddle on the floor, tears choking me.

I whisper, "I'm sorry," to my lover.

He gathers me in his arms and I feel his sorrow caused by my condition. He tells me he loves me and I try to be strong but tears break through and I damn myself for being so weak. When will the cycle of madness end?

5/25/98

Birds sail through the
Morning clouds
As the sun burns a hole
Of blue in the sky.
Days slip by
And summer is here.
Money to earn at work
Classes to teach
Books to sell.
A synopsis to write –
Just a page or two
To put the Rama book
In a nutshell.
Sleep calls me,
Even after a cup of java.
Learning humility every moment,
I think of my strengths
And weaknesses and
Put things in proper
Perspective.

11/16/98

I know it is the <u>act</u> of writing that keeps my power up; writing is my line into Eternity. Yet I still put it off and avoid the process by putting people between it and me. How very strange!

Even now, with two hours totally free, I think of doing dishes and laundry, and even cleaning the bathroom. Having a clean house is important to me, but it should not be an excuse to avoid what I need to do.

In some way, writing is my Dharma. I have always known this, but have never quite understood it. What do I need to write?

Anything from the heart.

I write technical manuals for money, but this work does not satisfy the inner craving. I need something more.

I like to be funny and open when I write, but lately it's been hard to find that place. I like the pen on paper, and writing at a computer is cool too. It's great when the words naturally flow.

On paper, I sell only 20 hours each week to my client; but in reality it is much more than that. My body takes so much longer to do even the simple tasks than it used to before this illness hit me. It wouldn't be fair to bill A&E for the extra time because it is my problem. It's the best job for this moment in time, so I will hang onto it for as long as I can. Sometimes I wonder if they will give my projects to someone else...they haven't given me anything new in months.

I can hear the helicopters searching the coastline. I hope they find the lost soul that was taken by the sea. When the ambulance went by, all the neighborhood dogs joined in the howling. Perhaps it was loud enough for the surfer or tourist to know help is on the way. It's amazing how many people fall off the cliffs. The jagged rocks and slippery sand must look inviting to some strange souls wandering by the sea. The helicopter sounds like it's circling round Point Loma where the surfers all hang out. The waves were small today; or so I heard on the radio. The fog is still sitting on the ocean like a white mist hiding the waves from me.

Whether or not the world is fascinating seems to depend upon your approach. When the world seems dull and boring, how do you change your approach? How do you move from not caring to caring?

Writing seems to help with this transformation. I feel it every time I let the words spill out, even if they don't make sense to anyone. Expunging the energy, the stuff that flows all around and within. Putting it on paper creates distance and makes it easier to be objective. Nothing matters. Only this moment is real; and then it's gone.

I also feel it happen during meditation; well, actually, it's more accurate to say I notice the transformation after I'm done meditating. When I'm feeling unmotivated, it can be difficult to remember that meditation works. The writing appears more immediate, to the ego anyway.

11/17/98

As the sun sets, a new life begins.
Twilight —
The moment before the stars shine.
Fog builds along the coastline
and swallows the sun as He travels west.
The ocean fills the crevices and cracks in the cliffs.
Water wearing down the sand and rock,
pushing the coastline a bit here and there.
Like a feather brushing across the land,
the roll of waves ripples the beach.
Pebbles and shells dig into the sand,
carving channels for the water to drain back into the sea.

12/2/98

Fighting sadness and despair left over from the Thanksgiving holiday. Jim brings me chocolate kisses to help break down the frozen wall of sorrow. The final A&E project is almost done and it forces me to look at future possibilities.

I wish they didn't take away the website project, but I do understand that they have to give the work to people who can do it in a reasonable amount of time. I've been fooling myself to think my managers haven't noticed the poor quality of my work. I want to do the work, and I would like to fight to get all of my projects back, but I don't have the energy. My body simply will not cooperate, and that frustrates me immensely.

~~~

Sorrow dissolves in the light of love.
Every day is a new adventure.
Perception of endless possibilities
Spinning through the Mind
Dancing on the edge of
Manifestation
There are no limits
There is no fate
There is only Love

3/5/99
Surrender.
Put it ALL on the table and offer it to Eternity.
It's not mine, never was,
So it's not too hard to give it back.
All these experiences,
         these feelings,
         these thoughts
They belong to Eternity.
I am not important.
I am merely a passing phase
Here one moment, gone the next,
Forever dancing in the light.

3/29/99

Reality slap 10 million 636…

My body is sick and it refuses to be ignored any longer. I've been putting this pain off for over a year: hiding it, making excuses for it, lying about it. It's time to deal with it.

I am tired yet alert, and the back of my head feels as if it's been hit with a bat. My back is all twisted and the burning, stinging pains shoot down my left shoulder, arm and into my hand. My neck keeps popping and my jaw won't open more than an inch, and even then it's puffy and stiff. Chewing is pure torture. One minute I'm freezing cold, and the next I'm burning up with the palms of my hands turning bright red.

All my pain and sorrow is released into the earth and sea...

Now if I could only look over my left shoulder without wincing in pain!

I release the pain, and start over again...

4/12/99

One year ago
I gave up.
(My heart went numb)
I let the pain of my body,
With the fevers and headaches,
Take control.
I stopped fighting
When my shoulder came out of its socket
and my hands went numb.
I gave up
When my jaw swelled to the size of a golf ball.

My time of mourning
Is over.

I gave up the Warrior's stance
When my Teacher died.
I let the pain of death
Envelop me.
Death is on the left, he said.
I watched helplessly
As the left side of my jaw
Swelled.
I cried helplessly
As my left shoulder fell out of joint.

Some small spark kept going,
Seeking answers,
Seeking healing.
Body workers pounded
Me back into shape.
Doctors gave me drugs to try.
Mourning for my Teacher,
I did not care.

Eternity gave me
A Task:
Teach, Open a Center.
I did
With that tiny spark of Light.

Still, my body ached
With pain
With fear

Burning with fever.
My Teacher said I could not
Follow when his time came.
I tried.
I wanted to lie down,
I died.

My contract ran out
My mind in a blur
Except
When teaching those things
My Teacher gave to me.

I sit now,
On sandstone cliffs
Facing the Pacific
Where I sat
Ten years ago
On an April day
Knowing
I am alive, in the world
And I must work, in the world
Despite the pain,
Despite the fear
Of falling.
I must get up
And find a way
To pay the bills.
My time of mourning
Is over.

4/25/99

Strength and weakness
Folding over and over
Cycles of motion and stillness
Clarity and forgetfulness
Bliss and suffering
Oily fish frying, stinking the air
Puffy white clouds give
Depth to the endless blue sky
Parrots fly by, grouped together
Safety in numbers.
A blue and gold Macaw finds a friend
Leaves dance in the gentle wind
In the wind, riding on the back of Jim's Harley, my hair flies.
My arms not yet strong enough
To ride my own bike, I settle
For what I can do: Hang on.

5/21/99

Body – what do you have to teach me?
What can I learn from this pain?
That all suffering is subjective and relative?
How do you wish to be treated?
What can I do to relieve the pain?
What do I need to do to rise above suffering?
How must my life change to accommodate you,
oh precious human body?
What do you need to express?
How can I show you love, embrace you in light?
What must I do for you to heal and be as One with Light?

Feelings fragmented by flashes of pain and
a few constant aches.
The body fights the mind's
relentless push upward.
Stopping the mind
Breathing the body
Visualizing pink light
Encasing the body,
Absorbing it in love
There is no fear here
Only peace.
The explosions of pain
Are like firecrackers,
Loud flashes
Leaving silence
As the light continues to penetrate
the core of every cell.

7/8/99

A cloudy, humid day with a few sprinkles escaping the sky. My body wracked with pain, even after an hour nap. Dealing minute by minute, day by day. Remembering all that I love. The scent of flowers and the earth. Jim and his touch, the feeling of our bodies pressed together. His smile. Meditation and the bliss that enters into me when I enter into timelessness. Rama – his light, his jokes, his love. Words on the page, how they fall and fit together, painting a picture. Spaz cat and the way she brushes against me, how she purrs when I scratch her chin. My family and friends, their smiles and comforting hugs and words. And of course, the ocean, the sun, and all of Mother Nature…

Balancing on a strand of Light,
Painted bright with love,
I dance alone.
Far below are the dark pits
Of anger and depression
Above are dreams that
Twinkle like stars at twilight.
This golden strand stretches
On forever behind me and
In front of me,
Always twisting and turning.
Next to me is my lover
We hold hands for a moment
Two souls on two infinite strands
Becoming one
For a timeless moment.
Separated we continue forward
Balancing all we know and love
Until we join again.

9/30/99

        Learning to accept pain without suffering... Bliss is our natural state. Beyond the body yet within it. Pure wonder. No judgments. Amazement.

        We fool ourselves into thinking we need a reason. A reason for everything. A reason to be happy? Why? If we quiet the mind and let the thoughts become quiet, we can feel bliss. It's always there.

Radiant Light
Beneath the surface yet flowing
Through all surfaces

Is pure radiant light
We are floating in it like a vast ocean
It is us.
Colored light merging and separating,
Undulating and swirling
Each wave unique
Lasting only a moment
Before dissolving
And forming
Into a new wave
An endless sea of waves
In ten directions
Radiating
Through the smallest drop to the largest sea

12/2/99

Pain sucks. I try not to resist the sensation. I try not to cringe as a thousand knives are stuck into my body. I try not to get frustrated when I can't spell or remember what I was about to do. I don't want to cry about it anymore.

How do I transcend pain? What does it mean to transcend pain?

Sometimes I can see past it. Sometimes I can do things despite it, but then I pay for it later. So that's not it.

Exhaling anger. Anger for not being healthy. Anger for not being able to do so many things. Anger for the pain I feel in doing the few things I do. The anger is rooted in attachment. Attachment to who I used to be. Who am I now? What role must I play?

The beautiful Spaz cat, preparing for her nap. Maybe I should take naps instead of trying to sleep through the night. I must have woken 10 times last night. Strange dreams where I was oh so sad and on the verge of giving up. I've felt that way lately about this pain; sometimes I want to give up and stay in bed. But that would make the pain worse. So I continue to fight for my mobility.

Sugar seems to help, but I wonder about the long-term effects, and it wears off too quickly. I must think of the things worth living for: time with Jim. Dharma Center. Enlightenment. Writing stories and poems. Laughing. Walking by the ocean.

It looks like this pen is dead...but I'm not.

12/7/99

Tears of sorrow
Tears of rage
Tears of loneliness
Of a life lost to pain and suffering
Why must this be?
Why can I not gather my strength
And heal this body?
What must I learn from this experience?
Why am I crying?
Today is no different than yesterday.
There was pain then just as there is now.
Yesterday I was strong
Today I feel beaten down
I want it all to go away
Why won't this pain stop?
Where does it come from?
What does it want from me?
How can I live like this?
Today I do not want to live like this.
And that frightens me –
The only escape route I see is death.

And that is too high a price to pay.
There must be another way.
Oh Lord, I am so tired.
Even my sorrow feels empty.
I feel so alone with this burden of pain.
I'm always wearing a mask, telling people it's not as bad as it really is.
I feel like I'm getting weaker –
How could I get any weaker?
They say Fibromyalgia is not progressive.
And so I worry that it's something else.
With all their medical knowledge
Why can't they tell me what's wrong with my body?
So many tears for so much lost time.
I don't know how long
I can go on like this –
Something's got to give.

1/4/2000
Write from the heart!
Find Joy wherever you happen to be.
So deep inside is the most tender spot
Touch it and it quivers –
Pleasure? Pain?
Something beyond
All of this.
No matter the mood, foul or fair –
This spot is the same
And there is comfort in the sameness, the equanimity.
This spot – this unmarkable space –
Feels like Love.

7/8/2000

In the darkest, tear-stained moments,
God is there.
In the lightest, ecstatic moments,
God is there.
Innocent unconditional love.
All you need to do
Is let go
Let go of fear, embrace courage
Let go of anger, embrace understanding
Let go of hate, embrace love
Let go of your self
And stop doing
Embrace being
Be infinite awareness
Be love
God is there
Waiting.

8/11/2000

Grasping the wish of health, I cringe in pain.
A sigh and a slight smile, I know
pleasure and pain are the same
Just feelings
Erupting
In the silence of the mind
OM MANI PADME HUM
(the jewel of Enlightenment is within the lotus of the heart)

1/2/01

Another new year, and the fight to heal continues. Wanting to sleep, but the z's don't come. Exhausted but awake once again. Everything seems so loud at night, after midnight. So how can I use this strange body stuff in my quest to follow Dharma and discover Enlightenment? Maybe listen to a Rama lecture? Or meditate some more? My body hurts from going all day long. I should be sleeping, but I'm not. Oh well, c'est la vie.

Relax. Relax. Relax. Why do I feel so wired? Must be the adrenaline from pushing myself. I have to get better at pacing. It seems like I can go for 45 to 60 minutes, and then I need to rest. Instead I've been pushing it to 1½ or 2 hours and then collapsing. I should know better by now. Yet I have no patience. I want to go, go, go.

Rhythmic snores echo from the bedroom, and Spaz cat lays stretched out on the living room floor, as I fill the blank pages with black squiggles of thought.

There was a time when I could sleep anywhere, anytime I felt the need. I could curl up on a couch, the floor, or even a sidewalk, in the middle of a party or in the silence of an empty house. Now sleep eludes me, hides from me in the sound of distant waves crashing against the shore.

Am I sad? No, quite the opposite despite the woes of my aching and sleepless body.

I feel alive and can smile with genuine joy – There is light in even the deepest shadows and there is love overflowing my heart. I am healing and I will sleep peacefully again someday.

9/26/01

Sleep is elusive tonight. A thousand and one thoughts roam through my mind as explosions of pain rupture throughout my body. Just another day on planet Earth.

Last night I slept some: I had a dream where I got shot with a shotgun and I died, and that's when I woke up from the dream. It was no big deal, even in the dream. It was like, OK I'm dead now, what else can I experience? So I went back to sleep in search of another dream.

A few hours ago Jim told me Jesse, Billy's wife, killed herself with a shotgun last night. We went to their wedding in July. I didn't know her very well and we talked only a few times. I remember she said she had really bad Endometriosis. So she was in a lot of pain, and I know from my own experience with the Endo that nothing helps with the pelvic pain. I wish she had talked it out with someone, instead of doing something so drastic, so permanent. Ughh. I hope Billy comes out of this OK.

Jim is very freaked out by it, because he's afraid the constant pain I face may make me want to do something like that too. I assured him there's no way I could I kill myself no matter how bad the body gets; I have too much to live for.

So now that makes three people I know who have blown their heads off with a gun. Two young women with shot guns and severe pelvic pain and one middle-aged alcoholic guy holding his depressed friend's handgun. What a waste. We get this life, in this body, only once. The details will never be the same, so why not make the best of it? To pull the trigger and throw your consciousness onto the Wheel of Karma with no guarantees you'll end up someplace better is not a choice I would make. My friend Mitch from high school left a note saying she was at peace with her decision, so perhaps she was in the best possible mind state to travel on the Wheel through the bardo and into a new life.

Maybe it's my own selfishness that clings to the pain of losing her and the others so suddenly. I feel Billy's sorrow so deeply because I know all too well the pain of losing a loved one in this way, when there's nowhere to put the anger.

*****

Life snuffed out in a flash
Of gunpowder and steel.
Ended – the torture of chronic pain
     invisible to others.
Ended – the love and joy of
     touching and laughing with another.
Here we are – trapped on this side
     in the world of seemingly solid form.
There they are – traveling on that side
     in the world of endless light,
Forgetting who they were as they
     return to this world in a new form.
It's all an ocean flowing forever
     between here and there and
     back again. Over and over.
We are the ocean – we remember
     for a moment, then we are lost
     in the boundaries of this droplet
     we call our Self.

8/20/04

The coffee is slow to brew this morning. Exhaustion weighs upon my body like the thick layer of clouds shielding the sun. I will my muscles to move and drag myself up to greet the new day. I want to run away from the aches, the pains, the cramps and spasms. But I know there is no where to run. Every moment I am shown the thousands of things I cannot control. In the silence I am shown the one thing I do control, the focus point of the mind. I choose where to rest my mind: beauty or horror, acceptance or helplessness, joy or fear. In timeless moments, absorbed in silence, I see beyond the duality and experience the endless, boundless bliss of Eternity. All of the frustrations from insurance companies and excruciating pain of the body are insignificant in the fire of Enlightenment.

Eventually I will learn to let go completely into Eternity's embrace. The "turning about in the seat consciousness" written about in the Sutras will transform the awareness of Self and my small mind will dissolve. Enlightenment will move this body of flesh through the world of duality, and shine the beacon of Truth, of Light, of God.

6/22/05
Grey sky brightens to blue as dawn approaches.
The full moon hangs low in the southwest
as I watch the coming of the light,
She is reflected by the windows,
appearing as three moons,
Watching and waiting with me.
The air chilled by night cools my hot feet, and
as the sky lightens, I cannot help but smile.

Take Action!

❖ Pick out a notebook for your own journal. It can be as simple as a school notebook of any size, or a fancy cloth bound book. If it's easier to type, use an electronic journal on your computer.

❖ Start your journal – grab a pen or keyboard and start writing! Write for yourself only; you don't need to share it with anyone. Give yourself permission to express your thoughts and feelings freely – bad grammar and all. Keep your journal in a safe place, so no one will "accidentally" read it. The pages are for your eyes only.

❖ Use your journal to record and release your experiences, both the happy and sad. The pages are for your eyes only. Let your mind wander onto the paper and perhaps you'll be surprised by what pops out. Most importantly, as my friend Milo once told me: "Write only what's on the inside, because it's cold out sometimes."

Meditation Practice

Breathe.

Rest your eyes on the period at the end of this sentence
and simply let yourself breathe.

There's no need to control the breath;
let it naturally move, in and out.
Sometimes fast, sometimes slow.
Let the body decide how much air it needs,
not the mind.
The body knows.

When the mind is too busy, it cannot hear the body,
nor can it hear Eternity.
Release conscious control of the breath;
trust the body, trust Eternity.
Watch and wait; do not touch the breath.

Within the silence,
there are layers upon layers of experience.
Let your perception shift and change with each new
layer. Don't cling to anything you feel, see, touch, hear,
or taste; don't run away either. Practice patience, and
let body and mind rest upon the breath.

Rest your eyes on the period at the end of this sentence
and simply let yourself breathe.

Breathe.

What Is Meditation?

Meditation begins when thought stops. It is silence. It is bliss. It is purity. It is peace. It is the awareness of that which lies beneath thought, emotion, and the physical world. Like swimming, meditation really cannot be described; it can only be experienced. Meditation is taking place right now within your being. If you quiet your mind, you will feel it.

Meditation is not the same as relaxation, although during meditation the body does relax. In meditation, there is an acute sense of awareness – it's like feeling everything at the same time, without being overwhelmed by it all. Within the meditative state, you are centered and calm.

Inside of your mind there is a still point from which all consciousness arises. Meditation is the practice of returning your focus to that still point. When the mind is centered in the stillness, there is silence, and beyond the silence there is unconditional joy greater than anything that can be experienced in this or any world. Beyond the bliss is the infinite depth of pure peace.

Meditation is the doorway to Light; it opens you to the Divine. No matter what your circumstances, when you dive into meditation and let go of conceptions, you will be free. Meditation is the way home.

Benefits Of Daily Meditation Practice

- Inner Peace

- Unconditional Joy

- Increased awareness of your Self and the world around you

- Increased energy and personal power

- Increased self-esteem and sense of well-being

- Ability to see and act on more opportunities

- Ability to use stress productively

- Stronger concentration skills

Preliminary Meditation Practices

There are probably more rituals and ceremonies that precede meditation practice than actual bare-bones meditation techniques. The rituals and ceremonies serve many purposes, with the most important (in my opinion) being that they help prepare the mind and body for meditation. A preliminary meditation practice may be as simple as lighting a stick of incense or a candle, or more complex like performing prostrations and reciting a short prayer or an entire sutra. Simple or complex, the intended result is the same: a calm, centered, grounded mind that slips effortlessly into meditation.

Focusing on the breath, without consciously changing it, is a practice that can be used anywhere, at any time. *Just Breathe* has become a cliché, yet there is truth to it. The real trick of the practice, that is – the hard part, is remembering to focus on the breath when your mind has spun out of control. Doing this can be especially difficult when well-intentioned people see you upset and remind you to breathe…it's almost as if the ego-mind takes this very good advice and creates more suffering with it. That shows you how twisted the mind can become.

The rituals we do before meditating, in essence, untwist the mind. If the mind is wrapped up in one tragedy or another, there won't be any room for the silence of meditation to exist. A bath or shower helps release some of the heaviness we carry both physically and mentally. The pleasant smell of incense helps reign in the mind's endless cascade of thoughts. The sweet smile of a Buddha or the intricate geometry of a yantra can hold the mind's attention long enough to break the train of thought. Reading a page of a spiritual book is yet another way to redirect the mind towards Light.

As you begin or restart your meditation practice, give yourself some time before each session for your own preliminary practice – whatever that may be.

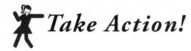 *Take Action!*

❖ Explore a few different preliminary practices, such as:

o Take a bath or shower. If you don't have time for that, then simply wash your hands and face.

o Stretch by reaching your hands out to your sides and up into the sky, then lower them in front of you with the palms facing each other.

o Light a stick of incense and pay attention to the aroma.

o Repeat a mantra, like Aum, seven times.

o Observe your breathing for a full minute.

❖ Create your own ritual from whatever inspires you.

How To Meditate

You can meditate any time, in any place, and it's free! There are literally thousands of meditation techniques available. Meditation techniques are a jumping off point to the silent mind. Most boil down to the same thing: using a focal point to stop thought. When you place all of your attention on one point, the mind becomes still, and eventually "you" go away in the silence.

It is simple, but not always easy. The concept of threading a needle is simple: you put the thread through the hole. However, if your hands shake and you cannot see clearly, this simple task becomes very difficult. The same is true for meditation. Focusing on one point is a simple task, but if your mind is jumping around, it is certainly not easy.

We begin with intent. We make a conscious choice to sit, with our minds and bodies still, for a predetermined amount of time. It may be as short as one minute; it may be as long as an hour. Stick to the time you set at the beginning; you can always sit longer if you want, but don't let yourself get up before clock runs out. I recommend starting with a short session of five minutes, and then gradually increasing the time. It is always better to have a short, focused meditation than a long distracted one.

In the very beginning, you are training yourself to

simply sit. It can take several weeks or months for your body to become accustomed to sitting still. So if you need to start with five minutes, or even one minute, that is a fine place to begin. The first step is to sit each day.

Once you have developed a consistent daily practice, increase the time to ten or fifteen minutes. When you're ready, increase the time again, perhaps to thirty minutes. After you're comfortable with thirty minutes, you can increase the time again, all the way up to one hour twice a day. It's always better to have a short, well-focused meditation session than a long thought-filled, spaced-out one. The hour is great, but only when you're ready.

Before sitting down, select a focal point. It can be a dot you draw on a blank piece of paper. It can be a flower, or a picture of a flower. It can be a Sanskrit symbol like the Aum in the Short Instructions at the start of this book. You may choose a Buddha, or a picture of Christ. Anything that looks beautiful to you is a good choice.

When selecting a focal point, do not use a picture of a person, unless you know without a doubt they are an Enlightened One, like a Buddha or Christ. You already have your own mind to deal with; bringing another person's mind into your meditation space only complicates things.

The focal point is your connection with Light, with God, with Eternity, with the Divine. Use something that evokes feelings of beauty and purity within you. Feeling that something is pleasant to look at is enough.

Another helpful tool is music. The music that appeals to you is an individual choice. I recommend using instrumental music in the beginning because music with lyrics can trigger thoughts. As you select music, pick something that evokes a bright, happy state. When exploring new music for meditation, I use the smile test. I plant a smile on my face and then turn on the music. If I can hold my smile while listening, I know I can use it for meditation.

Music can help blanket other distracting noises and provide an additional focal point. During each meditation session, you may find it useful to switch between focal points. For the first few minutes, focus on the visual object you selected. When that is no longer working, close your eyes and move your focus to the music. Switch back and forth as many times as you need to, keeping your focus on one or the other.

The music also works well as a timer. Instead of timing your meditation sessions in minutes, you can decide to sit for two or three songs.

Once you have decided how long and what to focus on, it's time to sit. As each thought or feeling or sensation rises in your mind, return your focus to the object you've selected. Don't fight the thoughts; simply turn your attention back to your focal point. Nothing else is important; only the focal point matters. Each time you pull your attention back, you are strengthening your willpower. Let go of the thoughts, feelings, and sensations – allow them to exist only in the background, passing by you and through you. As a thought captures your attention, release it by refocusing on the object. The only way to ignore something is to put your attention on something else. Ground your attention in your focal point until nothing else exists. Know that no effort is wasted; each time you pull back to your focal point, your willpower is growing stronger. You may want to close your eyes and visualize the object. When you become distracted, open your eyes and refocus your attention.

Be patient with your practice. In the beginning, it may feel like nothing is happening. Sometimes it may seem that you're thinking even more, because you're finally noticing how many thoughts are actually in your mind. It may take a while for the thoughts to slow down, and when they do stop, it may only be for a moment or two. As long as you put forth the effort to focus on one thing for a period of time, you will benefit from meditation practice.

Once you've sat for the allotted time, end the meditation with a bow. Give it back to Eternity. Whether it was wonderful or horrible doesn't matter; what matters is that you gave it your best. The bow is your chance to thank Eternity for the opportunity to sit. Eternity is always meditating; only when we stop thought do we notice the bliss and light continuously flowing through us.

Here is a step-by-step list to start your daily practice:

Step 1

Decide how long you're going to meditate and stick to it. Five minutes is a good length to start with; if that goes well, you can always sit longer, but don't sit for less time than you planned. Instrumental music is a wonderful timekeeper. The music creates a bubble around you, which helps to block out distractions. The everyday noises of the world become part of music, freeing you to stay focused. If you don't have access to music, use an alarm clock or kitchen timer. It's very difficult to concentrate if you keep looking at the clock wondering how much time has passed.

Step 2

Pick one thing to focus on. You can use anything that makes you feel happy or peaceful when you concentrate on it.

Some examples:
- Gold light surrounding your body
- A dot drawn on a piece of blank paper
- A flower or plant
- Buddha or Christ
- A pretty rock

Do not focus on people. You have your own mind to deal with and that's enough. When you focus on other people, you can pick up on whatever mind state they happen to be in at that moment, and it may not be a fun one. The only exception is an Enlightened Being, such as a Buddha or Christ.

Step 3

Sit comfortably, in a chair, on a cushion, or on the floor. Keep your back as straight as is possible for you. You can lean against a pillow if your back muscles are not strong enough to support you. Ideally, your shoulders should be straight and your chin should be parallel to the floor. Sitting cross-legged on a tall firm cushion can help to naturally align your spine. Put a blanket under the cushion to give your ankles some padding. The most important point about posture is to sit up and be comfortable. If you become horribly uncomfortable during a meditation, adjust your position without thinking about it too much. If your feet fall asleep, find a different position that does not cut off your circulation. You'll need to experiment with cushions or chairs to find what position works best for your body.

Don't lie down! Laying down makes it very difficult to meditate because your body becomes too relaxed and you may fall asleep or space out. However, it is possible to meditate lying down if you are experiencing a sufficient amount of severe pain, because the pain will keep you awake.

If you absolutely cannot sit up because the pain is too intense, try one of these positions:

1. Lie on the couch with pillows supporting you and sit up as much as possible. Only meditate in bed if absolutely necessary, since your body will want to fall asleep as soon as you begin to relax. Keeping your knees bent can help make you more alert, and provide a place for you to hold a picture to focus on.

2. Lie on your back on the floor with your knees bent. Rest your elbows on the floor and hold your hands in the air above your belly or chest with the tips of your fingers touching lightly. Pick one spot on the ceiling to focus on. As you meditate and quiet your mind, pay attention to your fingers: when your focus is too tight, they will mash together. When your focus is too relaxed, your fingers will separate. Keep

adjusting the intensity of your mental focus until your fingers are barely touching.

Step 4

Concentrate on your focal point, then close your eyes and try to visualize it. As thoughts arise, let them pass by like birds in the sky. Completely ignore any thought that comes up. Each time you find yourself distracted, gently pull your focus back by looking at your focal point. Let the thoughts come and go without concern. Focus.

There is a certain amount of effort involved, but don't try to force anything. You'll only frustrate yourself. Instead, remind yourself that you have nothing to do right now except sitting.

You can also use a word to pull you back; the instant you notice you've become lost in thought, let go and gently say "Aum" or "focus" or "light" (or whatever) to yourself and return to your focal point. You can say it out loud or silently.

As you sit, begin to notice the space in between the thoughts. Continue to bring your attention back to your focal point.

When the thoughts stop, surrender to the moment, to Eternity, to God. Completely let go of everything, including your Self. Trust Light.

Step 5

At the end of the meditation, it is customary to bow for a moment. This is your chance to say "thank-you" to Eternity. After all, it's not really you who meditates; all you're doing is getting out of the way of what is always present. The bow also helps to ground you, and it's a nice stretch after sitting.

 Take Action!

❖ Decide how long you will spend each day meditating, and stick to it for a week. If you find yourself getting squirmy or avoiding meditation, shorten the time. If it's easy to sit for that amount of time, try increasing it.

❖ For the most benefit, meditate twice a day. After you wake up (take a shower, drink some coffee or tea, stretch, etc.) and before you get involved with your day, give yourself some time to sit. Then in the evening, wash your face and sit again. Sunrise and sunset are especially wonderful times to spend in meditation.

Using Pain During Meditation

Sometimes the pain we experience becomes too intense to ignore. It takes over our consciousness until we are aware of nothing else. At moments like these, use the pain as your point of focus in meditation. When you are engulfed so completely by pain and screaming is not helping, you can do nothing else – so why not use it?

Accept the pain fully; do not run from it. This is difficult because we have been conditioned to retract from pain. That retraction is the body trying to protect itself; it is a natural response. Instead of fighting the pain, breathe into it.

Take a few minutes to do whatever you can to comfort the body, like lay down under a warm soft blanket. Stop thinking of all the things you wish you were doing. Your body wants your attention, so give it fully. Close your eyes and slowly scan your body from head to toe.

Watch your breathing. How does it feel when you inhale? How does it feel when you exhale? What does it feel like to be in between breaths? Does the breathing change as you focus on different parts of your body?

Pay attention to your body. What hurts the most? How does it hurt? Watch the pain. Does it move? Is it pulsating? How does the pain change from moment to moment?

Emotion and thoughts will try to push their way

to the surface. This is another way we retract from pain; the mind drowns us in emotion. If that doesn't work, the mind assaults us with thoughts and fantasy. Instead focus on the physical body. What does the pain feel like? Be fully present with it, with the body, right now. If tears flow, let them fall without judgment, without thinking about the tears. Let the body do what it needs to do, right now. Be present and wait.

As you sit with the pain, the attitudes you have towards your body may surface. Acknowledge and accept each one, and then return your focus to the body.

Over the course of many years of sitting with my own pain, I have faced a variety of attitudes. The feelings I held towards my own body included: despair, frustration, hate, betrayal, anger, fear, sorrow, guilt, shame, apathy, gratitude, joy, and finally love. The attitudes we have towards the body color our perception of it and of ourselves. Once we acknowledge and accept them, we are free to let them go. In the letting go, we realize we are not those attitudes. We see what we once thought defined us was really only a passing phase.

As you sit with your body and the pain ask, "Who is feeling the pain?"

You are not the pain. You are not this fragile body.

Inside of the pain, at the center of your being, there is a still point. There is an observer. And beyond the observer and the body being observed, there is the eternal you. That is where God lives.

Sit with God, with Light, with your True Self, as the transitory experience of pain passes through this world. Rest here. You will know when it is time to move again.

LET PAIN BE YOUR TEACHER

O great explorer,
Why do you quiver with Fear
In the face of Pain?
All your travels have shown you
Pain and Pleasure are transitory—
Ever moving, ever changing,
From one to the other
As the coin flips over and over
As the Wheel of Life turns.
Experience the pain of the body
With detachment.
The Eternal is beyond all Pain and Pleasure.
Know this and be Free.
Accept the 10,000 things as they are:
Illusions for your entertainment and education.
Hold onto nothing and be supported
By the Eternal.
Let Pain be your teacher.

What have you to show me, King of Pain?
There is no running away—
You will run only in circles,
Always returning to Me
Until the lesson is finished.
What must I learn from this experience?
Why is my body tortured when I eat?
Food is nourishment for the body; why does it come
with pain?
How can I remove the restrictions that prevent my body

from enjoying the nourishment it needs?

How do I open the channels of communication so I know what the body needs to grow?

Years of denying the Good of the body can be washed away in an instant.

Love the body unconditionally.

Respect the limits of the body.

Inhabit the body, for it is the vehicle of this world.

Make peace with the body and allow it to be your partner in the dance of Life.

There is no need to fight, no need to subdue or conquer the body.

Allow it to live in Light, in harmony with all aspects of your being.

All parts of being have the ability to perceive.

All parts of being have Power.

Trust each part to do its own work.

Maintain cooperation on all levels.

Understand one part cannot grow without the other.

Listen instead of commanding.

The physical body knows how to take care of itself.

The astral body knows how to take care of itself.

The Eternal knows how to be.

Let go of pre-conceived ideas and

Allow Life to happen.

Allow the Creative to move through the world.

Allow the Eternal to be all it is.

Inner Light

Everyone has within their being a spark of Light. This light is pure bliss, ecstasy, and perfect love. It is our true nature. Some have named it Christ-consciousness or Buddha-nature. This light is eternal and infinite and nothing can destroy it.

For most people, this inner light is a small spark buried beneath thick layers of conditioning, misunderstandings, and other pollution caused by ignorance of our true nature. Many people feel the inner light only during special times, like when watching a sunset, dancing with someone they love, or when a stranger shows them unselfish kindness. And there are some people whose light is covered so deeply they have no idea it exists. For them, life seems harsh, cold, and pointless.

The good news is the inner light is eternal. It is and will always be waiting – no matter what you do or think or feel.

Each time you meditate, the inner light grows brighter. Meditation and other spiritual practices feed this light, re-affirming the unity of the Creator and Creation. As the light brightens, it burns away the thick layers that cover it and pushes out towards the surface. Just as a pimple swells and pushes the infection out through the skin, the light pushes the impurities to the surface of our being so they may fall away. At times, this process may be uncomfortable and frightening. The body may react with crying and a variety of unpleasant feelings. Allow your tears to wash the impurities from your being and continue to focus on light, beauty and gratitude.

As you move through the purification process, it is important to forgive yourself and others for the suffering you have experienced. When a memory or image of who you once were comes up, consciously acknowledge it and let it go. The past is gone and cannot be changed, so indulging in self-pity in any form won't do you any good. Instead, honor your inner light by using your will power to make choices that bring more beauty into your life. Your body-mind structure is a sacred temple, and should be treated as such. You may make the same mistakes again and again. This is part of the learning process. Each time you make a mistake, learn what you can from it, and return to the Light.

It is only when the impurities reach the surface that they can be released. So when you discover the dark corners within your being, shine the light in them and smile. Laugh at your personal history and know it is only a distorted reflection of your true self. Strive to know the inner light by entering the silence of meditation. Ecstasy, bliss, and unconditional love are waiting…

Take Action!

❖ Sit in silence or with soft music for a full ten minutes today, practicing meditation.

❖ Throughout the day, once an hour, check in with your body and mind. Try to feel the inner light for a moment or two.

A Space Of Your Own

Most Americans have an area in their home for watching television. They have a nice television set equipped with cable or satellite and a comfortable couch. Once they sit down, the urge to flick on the tube rises, and most people do it without even thinking about it.

If you have a dining table you regularly eat at, you may have noticed hunger when you sit there at other times of the day. Maybe you didn't even notice it: you sat down at the table to write out a few checks and the next thing you know you're reaching for a cookie.

Most people would agree they experience some degree of sleepiness if they lay down on their bed in the middle of the day.

The body and mind each have a memory of their own. Connections to activities are formed when we do the same thing in the same place every day. This is why sleep experts agree your bed should be reserved exclusively for sleeping, with the only exception being sex, of course. The same reasoning applies to students: if given a specific place to do homework, they are more productive.

Because your body and mind remember what they are supposed to do in a given area, a dedicated meditation space is a wonderful gift you can give yourself when beginning or returning to daily meditation practice.

It is true – you can meditate anywhere, at any

time. However it is *easier* to meditate in the special space you have set aside for your practice. After a few weeks of daily practice, your mind will learn to quiet down and your body will automatically enter into relaxed attentiveness once you sit down on your meditation cushion. Over time, the psychic energy of every person who has ever been in or through that area will also clear away. Soon, you will be left with only your own thoughts to ignore during meditation practice…and that is plenty to deal with!

When selecting a place for meditation, it should be an area that will not be used for any other purpose. Ideally, it should have a couple of feet in front of it that no one (including yourself) will walk through. Look around your home for a rarely used corner. You may want to rearrange the furniture. Get someone to help if you need to move heavy items. The bedroom is an ideal room, since it's typically the quietest, but don't use your bed as your dedicated meditation area. Your bed is for sleeping.

If you have a small home, finding a meditation space may be a challenge. Be creative. Perhaps there's a table or chair you can pull away from the wall and you can sit behind it. A room divider screen can be used to block off a corner in a studio apartment so you're not looking at the rest of your life when you sit down to meditate. Really, you only need enough space for you to sit comfortably.

Reserving a space within your home for meditation sends a profound message to your Self, and to Eternity. It shows that the practice is important to you, and creates a physical sign that meditation is part of your life. Having the space already set up will make it easier for you to sit down, especially when you have only a few minutes. When you are having a bad day, your meditation area will remind you joyful peace is only a breath away. All you have to do is open to it.

Once you've selected your meditation area, clean it thoroughly. It should be spotless. If you have carpet, get out the crevice tool for your vacuum and suck away all the dust in the crack next to the wall. If you have hardwood, tile or laminate floors, wash it with water and high quality soap. Also wash the wall next to the space. Water neutralizes energy, and can help clear away any residue left behind by other people. Finally, use a stick of incense to help direct your will to clear the remaining energy. To direct your mind, use a simple phrase like: "This space is cleared of all energy; only the light of Enlightenment is present." You can make up your own phrase; just be sure to clear the old energy out <u>and</u> replace it with bright, clean energy. Visualize the space being filled with purifying light. Simply meditating in an area will eventually clear the energy; however these techniques will allow you to do it faster and require less personal power.

Purchase a new cushion or chair for yourself. If you cannot afford to buy something new, clean whatever you plan to use as best as you can. Don't use the cushion or chair for anything else; reserve it exclusively for meditation. Experiment with different styles of pillows, cushions, and/or chairs until you find the ones that let you sit up comfortably. If you decide to sit cross-legged on the floor, sit on a tall firm cushion. This will tilt your pelvis slightly forward, letting your back find its natural balance. Placing small pillows under your knees can alleviate the strain on your hips. Use a pillow to cushion your back if you need the support. Sometimes a small firm pillow between your lower back and the wall is enough to keep you sitting up straight.

Many people like to set up a small table in front of their meditation space with objects that inspire them. This is an excellent idea if you have the space for it. When you open your eyes, it helps to have something beautiful to look at. Use the table to hold your visualization object, or you may find it more comfortable to put it on the floor in front of you. Your table may have a picture or statue of a Buddha or Christ. Fresh flowers are wonderful, as are candles. Whatever helps you to feel Light is a good choice. However, keep pictures of people (unless they are fully Enlightened, like a Buddha or Christ) out of your meditation area. The table and the space are yours alone.

 Take Action!

❖ Pick out a spot now and try meditating there for a minute or two.

❖ If the first spot you picked doesn't feel right after a few days, try facing a different direction or selecting a new place to sit.

❖ Once you've found your meditation area, take the time to do a detailed cleaning.

Meditation Tools

Every good mechanic or craftsman has a set of tools. Tools improve our productivity; using the right tool makes the job easier.

Meditation is difficult, and more so when the body is screaming in pain. We can turn pain into a tool: it motivates us to practice, and it can be a focal point. Lots of people can tell you there is bliss and peace under the pain, but you won't know it until you discover it for yourself. All it takes is one moment of inner silence to feel the unconditional joy that is your true nature. Within that stillness, the pain of the body simply does not matter.

There are many traditional and not so traditional tools available to aid your meditation practice. We use tools to give the mind something to hold onto while we enjoy the stillness. During a meditation session, switch between your tools as often as needed. If one tool is not working at all for you, put it aside and try another. There is no "right" tool. They are merely devices to help quiet the mind so you can experience what is always there. Try out a few tools from the list below:

MUSIC

Have fun exploring the wide variety of artists in the music store, not just the ones in the New Age section. Instrumental music is best to start with because words can lead to concepts, and concepts lead to thoughts. As you become more comfortable meditating, feel free to explore any music that interests you. Some people enjoy soft, gentle music. Others prefer something with a faster beat. The important thing is to find music that feels good to you.

The test I use is to put a smile on my face, turn the music on, and see if I can hold the smile while listening. If I can, then I'll try meditating with that piece of music. Keep in mind that one album by an artist may work for you, and another by the same artist may not. *Tangerine Dream* is one of my favorite groups because they have an amazingly vast repertoire. I've included a list of some of my other favorite artists at the end of this book for you to use as a starting point.

Music not only makes a great timekeeper, it also provides an auditory blanket to cover up the distracting sounds of the world. Instead of labeling every noise you hear during meditation practice, you can let all the sounds become part of the music. The music can place you in a protective bubble, shielding you from the energy in your neighborhood. When you meditate, you can also focus on the music to hold your mind still.

BUDDHAS

Buddhas are real beings. Some have incarnated and walked the Earth as people, just like you and me. In fact, you are a Buddha; only you have not realized it yet. We call Buddhas "enlightened" or "self-realized" because they have come to know their true nature, that they are united with God. This is possible for anyone – if they want it more than anything else.

When using a picture or statue of a Buddha as a meditation tool, look at it until you can visualize it with your eyes closed. As you look into the Buddha's eyes, know you are looking into a perfect mirror and seeing your true self.

MANDALA

A mandala is an intricate drawing, sometimes consisting of geometric shapes and/or Buddhas. The mandala is a representation of the divine home of the various Buddhas. The practice is to memorize the drawing and recreate it in your mind with your eyes closed. This will strengthen your mind so you can hold more Light within your being and enter into very high states. When you have perfected the practice, your mind enters the world depicted by the mandala.

YANTRA

A yantra is a geometric pattern used to strengthen the mind, much like a mandala. Begin by focusing on the very center of the yantra; there is usually a dot there. After a minute or two, widen your focus to include the entire pattern. Keep your eyes soft; don't stare at it, instead gently gaze at the picture. As you gaze at the design, the lines may appear to move. Do your best to stay focused. After another five or ten minutes, close your eyes and see if you can re-create the image in your mind.

MANTRA

A mantra is a word or phrase repeated over and over, either out loud or silently within your mind.

Chanting helps to focus the mind and block out all distractions. This is an excellent practice, especially when you find yourself getting frustrated while out in the world. One of the most well-known mantras is the Sanskrit word Aum (OM), pronounced *"Aauummm."* Any word, phrase, or prayer that directs your mind towards God is a good choice. Experiment until you find a mantra that works for you, and then stick with that one. You can chant your mantra silently anytime to help you regain your balance, both on the meditation cushion and while interacting with the world.

Take Action!

❖ Sit in meditation and try switching between two different tools during your session. For example, chant a mantra seven times, then focus on the music for a minute. When your mind begins to wander, chant the mantra again. Then go back to the music. When you feel your mind become still, let go of the tool. When your mind begins to wander, pick up the tool again. Continue switching between tools until you reach the end of your meditation session.

❖ Create your own meditation tool. Perhaps there's a landscape photograph that makes you feel wonderful when you look at it... or a beautiful stone you found while out walking...or some other item that makes you feel happy when you focus on it.

Selecting A Meditation Class

There are many, many meditation teachers; however Life is the real teacher. It is constantly showing us the joy, the magic, the wonder of Light. Always remember: Life is the real teacher. Even if you have the blessed opportunity to sit with a fully Self-Realized Enlightened Being who is glowing with gold light and making you laugh hysterically, remember it is Life, or Eternity, using the form of that person to show you the Eternal Reality.

I encourage you to make every effort to explore the meditation classes available in your area. There are millions of teachers out there, sharing all sorts of liberating, interesting, and sometimes just plain weird stuff. Be open to learning whatever benefits you and your practice from anyone. Teachers sometimes show up in the most unexpected places.

If you are interested in Enlightenment – the real deal of Buddhahood – the path to Freedom, to know without doubt your True Eternal nature, then there are certain qualities to look for in a teacher. An Enlightened Being has two qualities: when they meditate they produce an unmistakable gold light, and they are outrageously funny. Some people see the gold light visually with their eyes; other people feel it within their mind; in either case it is unmistakable. You may find many teachers who have one of these qualities; however only the Enlightened will be both glowing and hilarious. This caliber of teacher is extremely rare in this world, but they do exist. If you truly need that level of teacher, you will find him or her.

To begin your practice, you do not need a fully Enlightened teacher. The tools within this book will get you started, and hopefully give you enough clarity to find the best class for you. Find the highest teacher you can who will accept you as their student, and then devote yourself fully to the practice of meditation and mindfulness.

It is not necessary to be interested in full, supreme Enlightenment to benefit from meditation practice with a group. Perhaps all you want is to feel better and experience more peace and happiness in your life. This is an excellent and achievable goal. A meditation class can help you develop the discipline of daily practice. Knowing others are also sitting on their cushions everyday can inspire you to sit when you don't feel like practicing. Having a friendly voice remind you to practice mindfulness can help you change your outlook from one of despair to joy instantly. With a meditation group, you can learn at your own pace and meet others who want to live brighter and happier lives.

While solitary practice is essential, there is a certain power in a group. The group consciousness amplifies the power of each individual, making meditation a little bit easier for the participants. Of course, this amplification can go either way; if the group degenerates into a moan and groan, complaint session then the people in the group will go down very quickly. Conversely, if the group discusses positive experiences, and uses the negative ones as learning opportunities then everyone can go up fairly easily. When one person gets stuck in their practice and then shares their experience, others can learn how to move forward along with the one who was stuck. A teacher or group facilitator will monitor the group and keep things on a positive and productive track.

The most important consideration in selecting a meditation class is how you feel afterwards. Check in with yourself about five or ten minutes after the class to see how you feel. Do you feel excited about your life? Are you happy? Do you feel inspired to practice? If not, figure out why. Is it your own resistance, or are you in the wrong class?

Once you've been sitting with a group for several months, make sure you are still progressing in the direction you want to go. Watching your own spiritual development is similar to watching your hair grow; unless your hair is very short, you probably won't notice the small daily changes. However, over time you can see that your hair has grown an inch or two. In the same way, if you look back over your journal entries you'll see what types of mind states you were living in three or six months ago. Then you'll be able to compare that to the mind states you're living in now. The questions to ask are the same: Do you feel excited about your life? Are you happy? Do you feel inspired to practice? If yes, then continue. If not, figure out why. Have you hit a block of your own resistance? Do you need to step away and practice alone for a while? Or is it time to explore a new group?

Finally, whatever you do, don't give up. Keep practicing, and keep looking until you find your tribe. It's important to have spiritual friends with whom you can spend time and who will understand when you discuss your experiences along the Path. Until you find your spiritual family, it's good to be low-key about your practice so those who do not appreciate meditation cannot discourage you. As the Buddha said, "It's better to travel alone than with a fool for company."

 Take Action!

- ❖ Go spiritual shopping. Explore the different groups who offer meditation as part of their practice. Be open and respectful of other people's views, even if you don't agree with them. If a group doesn't work for you, you can always leave.

- ❖ If you cannot find an existing meditation group, start an informal one with friends or neighbors who are interested in meditation. Break the meeting into two parts: a meditation session, and a discussion of a spiritual book or how you each are putting the practice to work in your own life. You may want to rotate the leadership role at each meeting to allow everyone to contribute fully. Always end the meetings on a positive note.

Meditation Tips

- Start with a short meditation session. You can start with 5 minutes or less. As meditation becomes easier or when it feels right, gradually increase to longer sessions by adding 5 or 10 minutes, up to 1 hour in the morning and 1 hour in the evening.

- Meditate at least once every day, even if it's only for a minute or two. This will help you build discipline and it gives you a chance to connect to the pure light and recharge your batteries. When you don't feel like meditating is often the time when you need it the most. **Sixty seconds of silence can brighten your entire day!**

- Find a spot in your house or room to dedicate to meditation. Clean the area and place a chair or cushion that you use for only meditation. Do your best to keep everyone else out of your meditation area at all times. By meditating in the same place, it helps clear the energy there. Psychologically it will build a connection that it's time for your mind to quiet once you sit down. Some people like to decorate their area with statues or flowers; use whatever you like that makes you feel good.

- Music is a very useful tool. It's a wonderful timekeeper and it gives you something to focus on. Pick something that lets you smile when you hear it. Start with music that has no words. Words lead to concepts, concepts to ideas, and ideas to thinking. Reserve your meditation music for only meditation.

- With all techniques, remember they are just tools to help you stop thought. If something's not working, throw it out and try something else. Visit different teachers and read different spiritual books to see what you can learn from each of them. Always trust your heart to know Truth.

- A good way to tell if you're sitting too long is how things look after you meditate. Wait a few minutes after the meditation and then just look around the room. Everything should look clear and sharp and you should feel peaceful or happy. If everything looks fuzzy and you feel spaced-out, you probably sat too long and let your mind wander too much.

- Never beat yourself up for missing a meditation. Instead, look forward to your next meditation. Try to build up some excitement and enthusiasm before you sit down to meditate. Say to yourself, "OH BOY, I get to meditate when I get home! YAY! I'm so excited!" Even if you don't fully mean it, talking to yourself in this silly way will at least make you smile.

- KEEP IT FUN!

Playing With Opposites

Sometimes the mind is too rattled to enter into silent meditation. You may sit down in front of your concentration object with the full intention of focusing until you can touch upon the stillness. However, the mind continues to interrupt you with what it believes to be very important thoughts. You put on music to quiet the world, you focus until you feel like you're going to explode, yet the mind continues to chatter on and on pulling you farther and farther into whatever particular state it has deemed so important. You've tried getting up and walking around for a few minutes, but when you sit back down, the chatter begins again. At these moments, it's fun to play with opposites.

Every state of mind has an opposite. That is the nature of duality. Before you can play, you'll need to put a label on your state of mind. Perhaps your mind is filled with frustration. I'm sure you have lots of interesting reasons why you have entered the room labeled Frustration. The reasons you're there are really not important. Your ego may want to go over all the reasons you are there, but just ignore those reasons for now. What's important is you know where you are. This will work for any mind state you find yourself in. For this example, let's use Frustration.

Stop everything for a moment and simply observe the mind state of Frustration. There's no need to judge it as good or bad or in any other way. Simply look at it and feel it.

Now ask yourself, what is the opposite of Frustration? Perhaps today the opposite is Acceptance. Tomorrow it might be something else, but for today, we've decided the opposite of frustration is acceptance. Take a peek and look at Acceptance. Once again, simply look at it and feel it.

At first, you may not remember what Acceptance feels like. To help you, use your imagination. Let yourself play with the idea of Acceptance. You don't have to accept anything in particular; simply allow yourself to experience what you imagine acceptance may feel like in your mind.

There's an ancient Tibetan practice called *tonglen* where you use these opposites to fully experience the dual nature of the mind. You can study tonglen in more depth through the writings of Jamgon Kongtrul and Pema Chödrön; however I'll give you enough to get started right now.

Take a moment to let go of any ideas that are attached to frustration or acceptance; simply focus on what those states feel like inside your mind. You don't need to be frustrated about anything, nor do you need to be accepting of anything.

As you sit there in the mind state of Frustration, breathe it in deeply. Feel it fully. Then, as you exhale, exhale Acceptance. Once again, as you exhale Acceptance, feel it fully. Continue breathing in Frustration and exhaling Acceptance. After a few minutes of breathing in and out, you will feel your mind shifting from one to the other. At this moment, you can choose to rest in pure Acceptance.

You have transformed Frustration into Acceptance with the power of your mind.

Now you are ready to practice silent meditation!

You can play with opposites any time you find your mind disturbed. You can carry the practice further by performing this taking-in and giving-out for others as well. Sometimes we feel helpless around people and animals who are suffering. What we can do very quietly is inhale their sorrow and send out joy with each exhalation. They may notice or they may not. It doesn't matter. It's an opportunity for you to face that particular pair of opposites and give selflessly to others. Each time you begin this practice, remember to start with your own mind, by doing the practice for yourself first, before taking in and giving out to the other person.

To take this practice even deeper, you can watch your mind swing from one state to its opposite and find the still point. Suppose your mind is trapped in pain. Accept the pain fully as you inhale. Then, as you exhale focus entirely on pleasure; use your imagination if you need to. Keep swinging back and forth, from a mind state of Pain to a mind state of Pleasure. Pay even closer attention to the middle point, in between these two opposites. With practice you can learn to stand here, watching the mind swing back and forth. This still point between the pairs of opposites is a doorway into silence. No matter what is going on, externally or internally, you can always rest here.

Take Action!

❖ Experiment with this technique right now. Examine your current mind state, and decide what to label it, and choose what its opposite is today. Breathe in your current mind state fully, and then exhale its opposite. Do this for 10 full breaths. (You can count on your fingers!)

❖ Try this practice at the beginning of your next meditation session.

❖ Before falling asleep in the evening, try it again.

Intentional Contemplation

In our life of chronic pain and illness, we often get caught up wondering why. The "why's" we ask about are not always about our health; sometimes they are about issues we would face even in a perfect body. We get stuck spinning around and around, trying to understand: why is all of this happening?

Well I hate to break it to you, but the why's are never answered. The why of everything is just a wonderful mystery with no concrete answer. There is always a deeper why. And sure, sometimes it's fun to sit and wonder why. But if we consider this quote from Tennyson: "Theirs not to wonder why / Theirs but to do and die" we see the truth of it. Even though you might come up with a really great theory of why something is, sooner or later something will occur that will blow your beautiful theory out of the water. So you can feed yourself the answer to why just to shut your mind up, knowing that you're just placating your mind. But deep down we know that we're really here to do and die.

Something much more interesting and helpful is to contemplate the what and the how. *What is making your mind react this way? How is it working?* With this approach, you have something you can actually do. You can sit there and wonder "Why is the world like this? Because people fight over power. Why do they fight over power? Because they like it. Why do they like it?" It just goes on and on and on and on, and you really don't get an answer. And even if you do eventually fabricate a conclusion about why a situation is the way it is, what do you do with it?

But if you look at the what: "What is going on and how it is working?" Then you have something to work with.

This practice of inquiring about the what and how of things is contemplation or reflection. The most common mistake of contemplation is approaching it as a quest for knowing why. Asking why can cause us to struggle and spin in a little circle over and over again. But contemplation or reflection is an important part of the practice, as long as you stay focused on learning the what and the how.

To give you an analogy, contemplation is the process of bringing you up to another view. So if you picture the path of spiritual growth as a big building and we're climbing to different floors so we can get a better view, you have two choices: you can take the elevator or you can take the stairs.

Sometimes when you're struggling with an issue, you sit with it and you contemplate it. You ask: "What is this issue?" Sometimes it's just a matter of getting in the elevator: you close everything else off, you're in the little box, just you and the thing you're contemplating, and it's pretty easy. You push the button and you wait and you look at it, because there's nothing else to look at except those four shiny walls, reflecting back at you. And you sit and you contemplate and then "Ding!" the doors open and you step out and you have a new view with these nice picture windows.

Other times it's more of a struggle; it's like climbing a steep staircase and you're dragging yourself up. It's this dark area with no windows, and you're trapped, climbing one step after another after another. And then finally you get it: you come to a resolution and you're able to open the door and see a new view.

What a lot of people do is they get stuck in the stairway. They forgot their keycard and they can't get out. They start questioning: "Why won't the door open?" And they stand there suffering until they realize what they need. Then they have to climb all the way back down the stairs and find the keycard. Or they forget to push the button in the elevator so they wind up going up and down, up and down, up and down, never figuring it out. Until maybe somebody happens to call the elevator and then *boom* you finally stop and walk out completely disoriented because you don't know what floor you're on – which can be a problem.

When you approach contemplation as a part of your practice, then you can use it to reach that next level. And again it's a matter of not getting sucked into trying to figure out why. Don't try to explain the mystery. Let it be a mystery. Enjoy that mystery, that sense of not really knowing why things are. But at the same time figuring out what it is and how it works.

So if you find yourself in your meditation or mindfulness practice, or in life in general, getting caught on the same issue over and over again, that's cause for contemplation. Create time where you're just going to sit, get in the elevator or walk into the staircase, and look at it. Look at that issue and ask "What is my mind doing? What is it really doing? How is it working? How is it processing this experience?"

Stop yourself if you begin to ask why, because that's our tendency, to figure out why I'm like this. You may decide, "Oh it's my mother's fault! It's her fault!" But even if it is, what good does that do? If you can instead say "What is my mind doing and how is it doing it? It's remembering how my mother used to react and I'm mirroring that." Then that's actually useful information you can apply and change your own perception.

The same applies when you're reading a spiritual book. If you're reading something and you're stumped or you have the other reaction, "That's bull! That can't be right!" Then it's always an exciting point to be at, because you're just on the cusp of a new perception. And sometimes your original perception actually is correct, that what you're reading is bull and the author was completely off or the translation was completely wrong. But in either case you come to a new understanding, a new view.

Intentional contemplation of spiritual teachings is a wonderful gift to yourself. Reading a small tidbit in the morning gives your mind something to chew on throughout the day. Spending a few minutes contemplating a teaching before your seated meditation can rein in the mind, making it easier to become still when it's time to formally sit.

Make contemplation part of your practice but watch out for the pitfall of obsession, of beating it to death over and over and over again. If you're not getting it and you're trapped on the staircase or elevator, that means you forgot your keycard and you've got to go back down to the lobby and work on your foundational practices of meditation and mindfulness some more.

Instead of contemplating an issue you're facing, write down a phrase or sentence to remind yourself of it. Writing it down allows you to let go of it and the worry that you'll forget it. Then practice meditation for 15 minutes. Once your meditation session is over, pick up the note you wrote yourself and slowly begin the contemplation process. Consider the what and the how of it. And then maybe when you're not thinking about it so hard, the resolution will come to you. The elevator door opens, "Ding!" And you can step out in that new view.

So practice your meditation and your mindfulness with that new perception until it's solid, and then something else will come into your field of experience that knocks you off balance and challenges you. Then you contemplate it and work on it and eventually that process will bring you up to yet another view. And then someday you might find a little railing that you look over and say "Oh wow, look at all that stuff I learned before!" That's kind of fun too, but don't fall over the railing. That's why there's a railing; don't climb on it.

This is all a practice, little by little. Like with anything, you can get lost in the obsession. There are thousands and thousands of philosophy books filled with explorations of the question why. It's an interesting diversion, and it can be fun once in a while - why is the sky blue? You'll get different answers from different people. Somebody might tell you "Hey it's not actually blue it just looks that way." And that may take all the fun out of it.

But I find it fun just to enjoy the mystery without

having to try to explain it away. When I catch my mind starting to wonder why, I have fun making up theories, the more ridiculous the better. I have a good laugh at it, and then I get back to work, back to practice.

 Take Action!

❖ Start adding some intentional contemplation practice into your day or your week. If you catch your mind tripping over the same issue, carve out some time to sit and fully concentrate on it. Meditate for a few minutes first and then actually contemplate "What does that mean? How is that working? How is it affecting me?" And as soon as that why comes up, stomp on it and push it out of your mind. Pull yourself back to the what and the how.

❖ Feed yourself some fresh mind candy once a day or once a week. Take just one line or concept from a spiritual book and focus on it throughout the day. Examine what it means to you, and how it applies to your life.

Meditation Recap

Seated meditation is the foundation of the practice. Without daily, seated meditation, progress is difficult at best. The seated meditation gives us the opportunity to simply let everything go. We can relax our body and mind, knowing everything will be waiting for us when we're done. While we are seated in the silence of meditation, we listen to our spirit and let it soar into the Light.

Sitting is not always easy; sometimes it's downright frustrating to even try to release all the things that weigh us down. In these cases, we use preliminary techniques to catch our mind and pull it back from its wanderings.

Before our formal seated meditation, we may wash our hands and face and do some stretching. Some days all we need to do is light a candle or a stick of incense and take a deep breath to quiet the mind. Other days, we need more.

If we feel stuck in a particular mind state, we may practice Tonglen, the technique of Playing with Opposites. We observe the mind state we are trapped in, and then we reach for its opposite. We allow ourselves to fully experience whatever mind state has us cornered, without judgment. We simply observe. Then we push the mind into the opposing mind state and fully experience that one. Slowly, we swing back and forth, paying special attention to the space in between the two mind states. Once the mind has become fluid, we are ready to begin our seated meditation practice. We focus the mind to one point, until nothing else exists.

Other times, we may find our mind gnawing on an issue that has knocked us off balance. We replay the scenario over and over, like a recording stuck on repeat. In this case, we use Intentional Contemplation to break the cycle. We write ourselves a note as an agreement to look deeply into the issue. Then we allow ourselves let go of it and sit in silent meditation for a few minutes, doing our best to hold still.

After our short meditation session, we calmly look into the issue and ask: "What is the mind doing? How is this happening?" When we are tempted to question why, we ignore it by returning to the issue and asking: "What is this really about?" We continue to dig deeper and deeper into our minds to find the root of the attachment that has us spinning in circles.

Once the root has been exposed, we can decide if it's worth holding onto or not. Even if we decide to hold onto that attachment, we understand what is causing the mind to circle and that knowledge allows us to take a break from it and meditate.

Playing with Opposites and Intentional Contemplation are supporting techniques for the practice of formal meditation. Use them as often as you wish; however they are not a replacement for the gift of seated meditation.

Sitting every day for at least a few minutes, doing nothing except holding your focus on a single point, is the most powerful thing you can do for your well-being. The rational mind may not be able to understand this, but you can prove it to yourself by devoting time each day to the practice.

The Mind

The mind is like the sky: perfect, clear, endless, and the container of all things. The sun may shine through the sky, making it appear to be blue. Clouds may fill the sky, making it appear gray. At night, stars twinkle through the sky, making it appear black. In reality, the sky is clear. It is only the coverings that make it appear blue, gray, or black. The same is true of the mind.

The mind is endless, yet we identify with whatever has temporarily filled the mind. When things go our way, we experience pleasure, and we believe we are that. When horrible things happen, we experience suffering, and we believe we are that.

You may be walking along in a wonderful mood when suddenly you stub your toe. For a moment, all that exists for you is the jolt of pain rushing through the stubbed toe. The world has literally shrunk to the size of your toe. The rational part of the mind jumps in, wanting to figure out what happened, and you become aware of the chair leg your toe hit. Slowly, the rest of the room comes back into your awareness field, and the toe continues to throb.

The typical person in this circumstance will indulge in that moment of pain, focusing on the throbbing. This will be followed by anger at the chair, and then anger towards himself or someone else, if he can find someone to blame for leaving the chair there.

The happy, wonderful mood evaporates into a mood of anger and frustration. This type of minor incident has the potential to ruin a person's entire day. That is how powerful the mind really is.

What if, upon stubbing your toe, you yell the customary expletive, make sure your toe is not broken, and then focus on the beauty around you? This would allow you to seamlessly go on with your day without giving the stubbed toe another thought. How different would your experience of life be if you acted this way in every unpleasant circumstance?

By learning how the mind works, and gaining control by focusing your mind on what you choose, you can dramatically change your experience of life – regardless of the circumstances of your body. The mind controls our perception of every experience. It creates the suffering we experience, and it is through the mind we free ourselves from the bondage of suffering.

The mind, by the act of perception, narrows your focus to a very small selection of possible experiences. For most people, this is an automatic process based on the training you unconsciously received from parents, teachers, and society. As you grew up, you were given a description of the world and without knowing the impact, you accepted that description. Within that description is a set of rules, like a computer program, which states if a certain thing happens, then you should have a certain type of thought. For example, if you stub your toe, then your thoughts should turn to anger and blame. As the program runs, you enter into different mind states and each mind state defines your field of awareness, that is, your perception of life.

Simply put, your mind has been trained over time to react the way it does. You have the power to alter that conditioning, to change how your mind automatically reacts to circumstance. The mind will continue to filter your experience of life no matter what you do; however by choosing the filter by controlling your mind, you can change and improve the programming and thus create a happier, brighter and more productive life.

Does this mean you can wish away your chronic pain? Perhaps, but probably not. People like to believe they (or others) have control over everything in the world. If you live in chronic pain, then you know sometimes you can't control even your own body, never mind the entire planet. While we can certainly influence the body and world by taking care of them to the best of our ability, if you've had any experience in the world you know things don't always work out the way you planned.

What you can control is the focus of your own mind, and in doing so you alter your experience of life in the deepest sense. You can live in chronic pain and at the same time feel joy, peace, and love. By directing the mind into these higher states, ecstasy and peace become the overriding factor and you can open to all that exists beyond the pain of the body.

You may think you live in an apartment or a house. That's just where your body lives. Where you live is actually in the mind, and it follows you everywhere. Or, as Dr. Seuss wrote: "Wherever you go, there you are." You can travel to an exotic island dripping with beauty and lavish comfort, yet your mind can linger on the horrific pain and all you notice are feathers poking out of the pillows and bugs crawling across the flowers. Alternatively, your body can be in the midst of a gallstone attack screaming in pain, while your mind rests in peace and your heart overflows with love. The pain is there; it's just not the main focus of your mind.

By recognizing the power of your mind and learning to harness it, you will have a better view of the opportunities available to you today. Instead of being a prisoner of whatever fills your mind, you can direct it towards light and fill it with beauty and gratitude. As your power develops and your awareness expands, you will be able to enjoy and appreciate each moment as it unfolds – no matter what life presents to you.

 Take Action!

❖ Stop for a moment and simply notice what thoughts are in your mind.

❖ Describe what mind state you are in right now. Is it happy, sad, excited, curious, or?

What Is Mindfulness?

Mindfulness is the practice of maintaining the contents of your mind. The Buddha said, "With our thoughts we make the world." Whatever thoughts running through your mind create the world in which you live. What kind of world are you creating?

Look inside your mind right now and see. Don't judge it as good or bad; simply accept whatever is there.

Those thoughts color your perception and cause you to act in a certain way, which in turn limits the opportunities available to you at any given moment. If you think someone is stupid, your mind will filter out anything contradicting the thought, and you will see only that person's stupidity. Everything to the contrary will be immediately dismissed by the mind.

Mindfulness ultimately leads to being fully present in each moment, without thought or judgment. We can simply experience what is happening now. This happens naturally when we are happy.

In the higher, brighter mind states we think less. Try to remember the last time you were engaged in laughter or another time when you were very happy. At those moments, you were fully present; all that existed was the now.

As you put into practice the teachings in this book, notice how many thoughts you have when you feel down, and how few thoughts you have when you are up. You can live in the higher mind states by learning to control the mind.

Through mindfulness practice, we train the mind by consciously selecting the thoughts that are helpful to us. Every moment we consciously choose which thoughts to focus on, and which ones to dismiss. The practice involves rewriting the automatic tendencies, which have evolved over years and years of conditioning. Eventually, we learn to use the power of the mind to see the world as it really is: an ever-changing fleeting dream, filled with magic, wonder, and mystery waiting to be explored.

Allowing unconditional joy to flow through you no matter what happens to or around you takes effort. It takes energy and willpower to stay in a high, happy state of mind, especially when the people around you are not and when your body hurts.

However, being unhappy and angry takes a whole lot more energy. Don't take my word for it; spend a day watching your mind and find out for yourself how much those unhappy mind states are really costing you.

Daily meditation practice will give you the initial burst of energy you need to begin practicing mindfulness. Your daylong mindfulness practice will strengthen your mind, keep your energy level up, and make your next meditation session easier. Mindfulness and meditation practice build on each other to help you develop a brighter, happier, more peaceful life.

Instead of being ruled by disturbing emotions, foul moods and distracting thoughts, you can choose a more positive and productive state of mind through the practice of mindfulness. All this requires is for you to make a conscious choice of what you hold in your mind.

Another way to phrase the Buddha's teaching is: WHAT YOU FOCUS ON YOU BECOME. So, if you *must* think, think happy thoughts!

As you begin to explore, it's important to realize we are sensitive to not only our own thoughts and emotions, but also to everyone else's, especially people we are close to, whether it be emotionally or physically.

Over time, you will learn which thoughts are yours and which ones are not. Spending time alone in nature will help you discover what your thoughts feel like. Remember, you can change only your own thoughts, not anyone else's.

In the beginning, mindfulness is much easier to talk about than to do. There are some baby-steps you can use to get started, and the benefits are felt quickly as you discover what knocks you off balance and burns up your energy. Once you learn your triggers, you can catch their effects early and eventually de-activate them.

Essentially, beginning mindfulness is a game of bouncing out negative thoughts by replacing them with positive ones. In the next section, you'll learn how to start playing the mindfulness game and discover for yourself how much the practice can benefit you.

Mindfulness Practice: Making Everyday Life A Meditation

Step 1

Pay attention to your thoughts and feelings without judging. Simply watch what happens within your mind and body throughout the day as you experience different types of thoughts and feelings.

Step 2

After you're comfortable with watching your thoughts and feelings, you may notice you have a little bit of distance from them. This distance allows you to exert some control over the state of your mind. When you notice a negative or unhappy thought, immediately focus on something positive. Beauty and gratitude are always available as ladders up out of nasty mind states. You can use anything that is available in the moment – a flower, a color, a nice car, a cool rock, etc. Use whatever you see around you and focus on its beauty as if it were the only thing in existence. Continue until you notice a shift to a more peaceful, happy state of mind.

The rational part of your mind may argue with you, justifying the negative thought pattern. Ignore it by returning your focus to the beauty in front of you, or to the feeling of gratitude you have for the things in your life at this moment.

Make a game out of replacing the negatives with positives. See how fast you can switch your perception from a downward spin to an upward spin. Look for and find the brightest side of every situation. Instead of focusing on the jerk who cut you off on the freeway, focus on how much you like the BMW he's driving and realize you wouldn't have seen it if he didn't cut in front of you.

Step 3

Bring mindfulness to all your activities. When you're involved in a task, put your full attention into every detail. Ignore any unrelated thoughts. Just like seated meditation, push away thoughts or feelings about anything other than the task you are working on. Ignore the thoughts by refocusing your attention on the task. Eventually, the thoughts will go away and the task will become a meditation. Do this all day long and you'll find at the end of the day you'll feel happy and energized, instead of sad and exhausted. Your body may be tired, but you won't have the heavy mental exhaustion that often goes with chronic pain.

Step 4

After practicing both meditation and mindfulness for a while, you may begin to notice times when you no longer need to think. This is being completely present, in the moment. You will be able to observe and enjoy life as it unfolds before you. You may feel a sense of equanimity and a sense of compassion for every living thing. Enjoy it all and stay active in your life.

Continue to start over at Step One every time you notice you haven't been practicing mindfulness. Even if you've been practicing for 10 years, start over at the beginning. Each time you pull your mind into a higher state, you have increased your willpower. While you may not notice the change immediately, your mind will grow stronger every day.

Remember: Meditation and mindfulness are a PRACTICE, not an accomplishment.

Smile Before Sleeping

Mindfulness practice is challenging. Without doing the seated meditation practice, it can be nearly impossible to pull up enough power to move your mind from the gutter of despair into the beauty and joy of light. There is one time of day when the practice is a little bit easier: just before falling asleep.

Once you've brushed your teeth and are ready to climb into bed for the night, you have already decided to stop for the day. Whatever issues are confronting you, whatever nightmare you may be living through, at that moment you have made a decision to let it all go and sleep.

As you lay there in the dark, just before you close your eyes, take a few moments to gain control over your mind. Consciously move your mind from the dark depths of suffering by focusing on gratitude or beauty or silliness. Give yourself permission to forget about your body, your life and your world, and dive into senseless joy.

You've already decided there's nothing else you are going to do today; you're already in bed, ready to sleep. All those thoughts of days past and days yet to come do not matter right now. Ignore all the thoughts and make yourself smile.

Do whatever it takes, whether it feels ridiculous

or fake or just plain weird. Plaster a big, fat smile on your face and hold it. Keep holding it until you cannot help but laugh at yourself. If you need to, get up and stand in front of the mirror. Watch your smiling face, and let yourself indulge in the silliness of staring at your big goofy grin in the mirror. Give yourself at least 5 minutes of smiling, and keep pushing towards the light until you feel yourself shift into a brighter, happier state of mind.

Repeat this every night, and always fall asleep with a smile on your face.

 Take Action!

❖ Why wait for bedtime? Get some smile practice in right now! Put a smile on your face. If you're having trouble, go stand in front of the mirror and smile for at least 5 full minutes.

❖ Try it again tonight, as you settle into bed.

❖ When you first wake in the morning, give yourself a little smile before getting up.

Using Karma To Your Advantage

Karma is the underlying force that causes us to perceive the universe in the manner in which we do. Many people simplify karma to mean for every action, there is an effect. While this basic definition is true, what people fail to take into account is the exponential property of karma. Every individual who is living (or has ever lived) produces karma through physical and mental actions. Each of those actions creates a wave of effects, radiating from every individual action. These waves of karma overlap and interact, and thus create the world in which we live.

When it comes to purely physical karma, we have only a small influence because of the enormity of the number of karmic waves. In other words, the physical karma we receive is not always a direct result of an action we performed; we may have merely been in the path of an ongoing wave that started long ago. If someone hits us with a car it does not mean we at some point hit that person with a car. How we handle the experience, however, is determined by our individual, mental karma.

Our personal karma actually has more to with the intentions and thoughts attached to an action than the action itself. It's the state of our mind that produces our karma, both good and bad. The accumulated effect of a person's karma will then create the overall level of awareness of an individual. The higher one's awareness, the happier, brighter, and more open and at peace one will be.

For example, if you are feeling very frustrated and irritated, then through the force of karma you will sink into a low state of mind and your awareness field will shrink. You will be more aware of all of the things that frustrate and irritate you than anything else. It's as if you create a magnetic pull towards things associated with that state of mind.

Perhaps you leave the house in a mind state of frustration. The rain has left everything soaked, and you accidentally step into a puddle. As you go about your day, you may find yourself dealing with an abnormally large number of annoying people who get in your way as if they knew you were feeling bad. At the store someone bumps into you, sending searing pain through your arm. You don't even hear the apology; all you feel is anger. Then you discover you cannot reach the box of cereal you want from the top shelf. It may seem as if the entire world consists solely of idiots.

On a different day, you may be in a state of happiness. (Maybe because you gave yourself time to meditate.) Your physical pain is present, yet within your mind you feel joy and peace. As you leave the house, you notice a tiny bird singing a beautiful melody. You stop for a moment to listen and you notice the sun sparkling in a puddle left by the previous night's rain. You step around the puddle. At the store, someone bumps into you, and even though it hurts, you accept the stranger's apology with a smile. You notice the cereal is on the top shelf, so you ask the stranger to pull it down for you.

Wherever you go, people seem to go out of their way to accommodate and help you.

By controlling the state of mind we live in, we control our karma. It's easier to maintain a higher, happier mind state than to move into one from a state of darkness because of the force of karma. So take heart, even though it may be difficult to find peace initially, it gets easier with practice.

When practicing mindfulness, pay special attention to how it feels to be in a peaceful, happy state of mind. Use the memory of those moments to inspire you work through the bad times. Also realize that every time you pull yourself up to a higher state of mind, you are contributing a little more brightness to the world. Even though the effect seems small, it creates a positive wave of karma for yourself and others.

Sometimes I hear people say, "Oh I have bad karma, that's why I feel so miserable." They speak as if they have nothing to do with their karma, as if it's somehow outside of their control. Your future karma is always within your control. True, if you've been indulging in nasty dark mind states, you will have to work hard to overcome the established flow. It's important to remember you created the direction of the flow, and you have the power to reverse it.

There is always a way out, no matter how bleak your life may appear. You always have a choice: to remain in misery, or work to move past it. The practice of mindfulness moves your mind from your bad karma (low mind states) and into higher, happier states, which translates into good karma.

As you begin to change your karma through the

practice of mindfulness, the residue of your past mind states will continue to arise as the waves of previously created karma crest. At that moment, you have a choice: to give into that past state, or push through it into joy.

It often takes time for the external circumstances of your life to catch up. If you have spent years trading complaints with a certain friend, then that friend will expect your conversations to continue to be a series of complaints. It will take practice to change the karmic pattern you have created with that friend; however by directing your conversations towards upbeat topics, eventually the quality of your talks will improve. In the meantime, you can use each situation as a challenge to push yourself into a higher and happier state of mind.

Improving your karma does not mean that everything will magically work out the way you want it to – although sometimes it does! What it means is because you are happier, your awareness is larger, and you will notice opportunities you may have missed before because you were in a dark place.

As you meditate each day, you will naturally over time develop a sense of non-attachment. At first, you may only notice that the things that used to bother you no longer do. This is the very early stage of moving beyond karma towards Liberation. If this is something that interests you, there are many excellent resources to explore. The titles of some of these books are included in the Resources section.

For now, an understanding of karma will help to improve your mindfulness practice. This understanding provides motivation to live as high as possible every moment of every day, no matter what is happening to your body or around you physically.

Karma creates the situations you experience, and influences your reactions to them. Your reaction, based on your current mind state will then create more karmic waves, which will then create the next mind state you experience and color your perception of the next situation, and so on. By being aware at the moment of reaction, you can draw upon free will. In this moment, you have the choice of whether or not to continue your current karmic pattern.

Meditation increases your awareness and strengthens your willpower. Mindfulness provides the presence of mind needed to make a conscious choice of how to react to the thoughts and feelings arising within you. Your reactions will then cause you to make the choices that create your perception of the world in which you live. These twin practices will give you the opportunity to use karma to your advantage, instead of being whipped around by it.

Take Action!

❖ The measure of how well you use karma to your advantage is not how long you can stay high. The real test is how fast you can turn it around when you start to sink into lower mind states.

❖ For the next five minutes, review the events in your life for the past day or week. Sit back and objectively watch what you experienced. Now ask:

  o Were there any moments where you were carried along by karma, stuck in an old pattern of behavior?

  o Were there any moments where you controlled your reactions and changed your karma for the better?

❖ Once the five minutes is over, let go of the past and focus on the present.

Fleeting Feelings Of Emotions

Fighting frustration and
Hypersensitivity.
Moments in time
Crash into the past
As seconds flash by.
Clawing my way
Up
Through the portal
Seeking
A deeper peace.

An emotion lasts for only a moment. The mind grabs hold of the emotions you experience with thoughts about the emotion. The mind considers why you're having that particular emotion, other times you had the emotion, and whether or not it enjoys the emotion. Then the memory of that emotion is played over and over in the mind through this thought process. In the meantime, you miss all of the other interesting emotions you may actually be feeling during those moments you are stuck in your thoughts.

Spiritual practice is not about denying and repressing unpleasant emotions. Many people look to meditation as a way to escape negative feelings. They confuse the practice of mindfulness (the practice of controlling and moving beyond thoughts) with controlling their emotions. Emotions cannot be controlled; they are fleeting. Emotions can be denied; however, denial is not freedom. You can fool yourself for only a short period of time. Eventually the disturbing emotion is experienced again, and the thoughts about the emotion take over.

Controlling and letting go of thought does not mean you will no longer feel emotions. Meditation is not an escape from feeling. Quite the opposite: without the obstruction of thought, emotions are deeper and richer. Imagine being able to love with your entire heart instead of holding back and checking yourself with thoughts about whether you or the other person deserves love. However, emotions last for only a moment – blazing through your being in all their glory.

When we experience joyful emotions, we tend to embrace the emotion fully. When we share a big belly laugh with someone, we feel it completely in all its wonderful intensity. Later, when we remember the feeling of laughter, we smile, but it's not as intense as the original emotion. We instantly recognize the difference between the genuine emotion and the memory of the emotion. That's why we don't usually get "stuck" in pleasant feelings.

Unpleasant emotions, however, cause us to turn away and hide because they are, well, unpleasant. We remove ourselves mentally from the experience, shielding ourselves from the full intensity. We still feel the unpleasant emotion; however it is muted. So even moments later, when the memory of that feeling rises, it appears the same as the original emotion.

During this instant re-play, we believe we are still experiencing the emotion, and not merely the thought and memory of it. Once again, we push it down into the shadows of our being, unaware it is only a memory that can be let go. We know we have only pushed it down, so eventually it rises again, replaying the memory of emotion, and all the thoughts that go with it.

Simply by recognizing that the original emotion is gone, we can let go of it and move the mind away from the endless train of thoughts triggered by that particular emotion.

Once we regain control of our thoughts, we are free to experience the new emotions appearing and disappearing at every moment. Emotions pass through us very quickly, sometimes like sudden storms and other times like a rainbow, which disappears in the blink of an eye. Enjoy the pleasant ones without attachment, and don't fear the unpleasant ones because they too will pass.

 Take Action!

❖ For the next three minutes, allow yourself to fully experience whatever emotions rise within you. Don't cling and don't pull away. Simply feel.

❖ Add the noticing of emotion to your mindfulness practice. Begin to recognize the difference between a true, fresh emotion and the memory (or thought) of an emotion. Remember emotions are fleeting; don't give them more weight than they deserve.

Don't Take Anything Personally

When most people have a bad experience, they assume someone is angry because of them, or the Universe is out to get them, or God is somehow punishing them. In other words, people have the tendency to take everything that happens personally. This is one of the biggest causes of suffering, and one that is completely avoidable.

We have been conditioned to perceive the world from this egocentric vantage point. When we cried as a child, Mother or Father would come running to help us. As we grow up, we realize there are other people, but we still want to believe we are the center of life, and anything others do around us must have something to do with us. In reality, most of the time how other people act has very little to do with us.

Our ego likes to believe we can control other people; we want to believe they have to come running when we want them. This perception makes us feel powerful and gives us a sense of connection with others. In short, it makes us feel important. Even when this belief causes unpleasant experiences, we hold onto it. When the cashier closes his line to go on break and tells us to go to another line, we become offended. Some small part of us actually believes he intentionally closed the line on us, and not that it was simply time for his break.

When we need a favor from a friend, we expect

her to help right away. If she doesn't, then we feel we must have done something to make her angry. We take her unavailability personally, when in fact her previous commitments had nothing to do with us. With the ego out of control, we spin into self-pity and ask: "Why won't she help me?" When our friend does arrive to help at a time that fits her schedule, we greet her with mixed feelings of resentment and gratitude.

In another case, if someone asks you for a favor, and you cannot do it, you may feel bad about not being able to help. You believe they will take it personally, and this sends you into a mind state of guilt. Or, you try to do it anyway and end up hurting yourself in some way, triggering a mind state of resentment towards the one who asked for your help. All of this suffering is because you take things personally, and you assume others do as well.

It can be tricky finding the balance between focusing on your own needs and remembering you are not the center of the universe. As you take care of yourself, it's helpful to keep in mind other people have needs to fulfill as well. Life will go on without you, yet you as an individual bring unique qualities to the human race only you can express in that particular way. So, yes you are special, but so is everyone else. Does that in any way diminish your special-ness? It does only if you view life from the personal, it's-all-about-me perspective. On the other hand, if you appreciate your own and everyone else's uniqueness, it becomes much easier to not take things so personally.

The next time you find yourself being treated rudely or in some other way you don't want to be treated, realize it's not about you. Whoever happened to come along would have probably received the same treatment from this person.

Of course it's difficult when the doctor you are seeking medical advice from treats you badly. It will feel worse if you decide to take his mistreatment personally. Instead, stop for a moment to consider how horrible the doctor must feel in order to treat anyone that way. Then, with compassion and diplomacy, express your perception of his treatment towards you. Sometimes doctors are not aware of how much their mannerisms and emotions affect their patients, especially the ones who are hypersensitive from constant pain.

It's important to understand many doctors become frustrated when faced with patients who have intractable pain, and this irritation can surface during appointments. The frustration has to do with the doctor's feeling of helplessness, and has nothing to do with the patient as a person. You can sometimes help the doctor overcome his frustration by expressing your appreciation for him doing his best to help you.

Occasionally you will run into people, including doctors, who are so miserable that the only way they know how to make themselves feel better is by putting others down. In these cases, remembering not to take things personally will help you a great deal. Obviously if you discover your doctor is one of these rare people and you are not able to resolve the situation, find another doctor to treat you.

Ultimately, you need to remember you cannot change another person. You can only control the focus of your own mind. You are entitled to a life of unconditional joy and inner peace; however you cannot force others to accept joy and peace in their life. By giving the people you meet the freedom to be however they happen to be that day, without taking their actions personally, you give yourself the power to open to your own depths of joy and peace.

 Take Action!

❖ Set your intent to see life from a broader perspective, where everyone is just as unique and important as you are.

❖ When you are around other people, watch your mind carefully. How does it react when others do not do what you expect?

❖ Practice being quietly happy, even when the people around you are not.

Dealing With Other People

*"Bondage and liberation, satisfaction and anxiety,
sickness and renewed health, hunger and so forth –
these are matters of personal experience.
You know yourself. Others can only guess at your condition."*
~Shankara's Crest Jewel of Discrimination

Interacting with other people is one of the most challenging situations a spiritual seeker faces; coupled with physical pain, this challenge is even more difficult. Humans are social creatures; so to live locked away without contact with others seals off a part of our nature. Even the monk who lives for years alone in a cave meditating eventually has to come out to test her enlightenment in the world. While spending time alone is useful and enjoyable, spending time with others is equally useful and enjoyable.

If you live with others and want to follow the practices outlined in this book, it's important for your housemates to understand you need to spend some time alone in meditation each day. It doesn't matter if they want to join you in practice or not; what's important is you give yourself the room to do your practice. Even if you live alone, give yourself this time by shutting off the ringer on your phone.

People need boundaries. Most people do not know how to act around someone who lives with chronic pain.

These well-meaning friends and family bounce between pity or sorrow and ignorance or denial of your situation. Each time you go out with friends, you may need to educate them on your needs. I have found I can walk longer if I go slowly; I often have to remind the people I'm with to slow down. If they don't listen, I simply walk at my own pace and let them go ahead; eventually they stop to wait for me. Another example may be when you visit a museum and you become tired, it's important to sit down at the first bench you see and explain to your friends you must rest. If your body gets stiff when watching a movie, pick an aisle seat and caution your friends that you may need to get up to stretch halfway through the film.

To those of us who live in pain, these small actions become second nature; to others they may seem strange. The feeling of strangeness is a problem for your friends to deal with, not you. You may be able to help them through it by explaining your needs, but ultimately it is up to them to work through it. If you let their feeling of awkwardness overwhelm you, you may be tempted to skip the little actions that make you feel better. The result will be your friends feeling badly because they think they caused you more pain, and they may not want to invite you out next time because they are trying to protect you. You need to teach them you know how to protect and care for yourself by respecting your limitations, even when they don't.

Subtlety is a lost art. Once upon a time, a person could drop a few hints and a conversation would naturally come to an end, or a friend would automatically offer a helping hand. In today's world, direct requests are welcomed. Be clear about what you need or want from someone and ask for it. Always provide a way for the person to turn down your request without feelings of guilt. More often than not, if a person has time to help you, he will. For example, if driving wipes you out, ask your friends to pick you up and explain to them how this will allow you to spend more quality time with them. If they cannot meet you at your house, then ask to meet them halfway. Compromise never goes out of style.

As your practice develops, you will become both more sensitive and stronger over time. This is your awareness expanding. At times, it may feel overwhelming because it can be difficult to sort out what thoughts and feelings are yours and which ones are coming from others. You may go to a support group one week and go home feeling positive and energized. The next week, you may go home feeling drained and depressed. It could have more to do with whom you sat next to, rather than how you actually feel.

Spending time alone, preferably in nature, is an excellent way to get in touch with how you feel, and where your thought patterns take you. You don't need to go on a five-mile hike; simply driving to a park and sitting next to a tree will work. The only catch is you need to go alone. Your home has the residual energy from all the people who have ever been there, so it's not as effective as going out to a park. If you cannot drive, then your backyard or any outdoor place will do.

Once you get to the park, simply sit and experience your Self. It may take a few minutes for all the chatter of thoughts to quiet down. You can try asking yourself: "What do I feel like?" a few times to help you focus on only yourself. Another technique is to bring a notebook with you and write whatever comes out. Examine closely the thoughts and feelings pouring out of you. There's nothing to judge; this is simply an exercise to see what is underneath all of the clutter. Repeat this often.

After doing this exercise, pay close attention to your mind when you encounter other people, and even when you arrive at home. Ask yourself, "Is this feeling or thought mine, or is it coming from someone else?" You may be surprised at how many of the thoughts you think are not your own. If it's not yours, then it's easy to push it out of your mind. You cannot change what is not yours, but you can easily let it go by recognizing that it doesn't belong to your mind. If you discover the thought is yours and it is not productive, then change it by focusing on the beauty all around you.

You cannot fix other people, just as they cannot fix you. Most people spend a great deal of time and energy carrying around other people's baggage. Your friend may feel better for a few minutes, but before you know it, she has picked up even more baggage. Over time she actually starts to expect you to pick up her mess, because you have always done so. Once you realize it's not your problem, you can let go and the baggage will return to where it belongs. Then you are free to work on your own issues and create your very own excellent life.

This may sound cold, especially when you find yourself in need of a friend's support, but really it's not; it's intelligent. Why carry around negative thoughts that are not yours when you can do nothing to change them? All you can really do for someone else is be an example of the peace available to us all by taking good care of your own mind. When you need support from a friend, call and talk out your issues, knowing at the same time you are the one who has to deal with them. And of course, always thank the friend for letting you vent. Verbalizing your gratitude at the end will make you both feel better. Remember, gratitude will always pull you up to a higher mind state. Then one day, it will be your friend's turn to call you and vent. If she forgets to thank you, you can say something like, "I'm glad I could help you vent." This type of statement also turns the energy of the conversation towards gratitude.

If someone calls only to use you and never helps you in return, then perhaps the next time she calls you could tell her you are too busy today. That type of person will move on to someone else if they can no longer abuse you. While those who solely abuse others are rare, they do exist. Allowing the abuse to continue hurts both you and the abuser by keeping you both stuck in a detrimental cycle.

There are billions of people in the world; if you make yourself available, you will find someone with whom you can build a true friendship where there is a fair exchange of help, gratitude, and joy.

If on the other hand, you discover you are the one who uses people up without ever offering anything in return, that's an issue for you to work on. Don't feel bad or guilty about it. It's simply an unhealthy habit you have learned. You can learn a new, higher way of interacting with others. Practice generosity and gratitude as often as possible. Let other people go ahead of you in line once in a while. Say "thank you" and dig inside your heart so you really mean it.

If you feel inclined, tell those close to you of your realization, and ask them to gently remind you when you try to take advantage of them again. For this change of behavior to happen, you must work very hard, each and every moment. Keep your eyes open for opportunities to help others in whatever way you can, rather than receiving it for yourself. You will find the giving is much more rewarding.

Dealing with strangers can be somewhat different than when you interact with friends and family. Unless you have an obvious sign of disability, the strangers you meet while out in the world have no idea of your physical situation, and they probably don't want to know. Even if you are in a wheelchair or using a cane, strangers still don't know the whole story. You may feel as if you are about to collapse from pain and fatigue, but no one else knows that by looking at you. You may be able to look in the mirror and see the dark circles under your eyes and the paleness of your complexion; to others you look normal. If you require special help, you will need to ask.

At the grocery store, ask for help picking up a heavy item like bottled water, or help taking your bags to the car. If I go shopping alone, I always ask them to pack the bags light, so I can take them into the house one at a time instead of struggling with a heavy bag. You really don't need to explain why you need help; in most cases asking is enough. Another example is when I stop to buy a small bottle of juice to drink; I'll ask the cashier to open it for me. Most people I have encountered are happy to help, and a simple "thank you" is enough to make them want to do it again.

When you visit your doctor, it's time to be honest

and completely spill your guts about everything you experience. The doctor's office is the one place where it's important to share all the gory details of your pain and how it affects your life. Your friends and family do not need to know every detail, but your doctor does. If you don't tell the doctor, he or she won't know and won't be able to help you.

When my illness was out of control, I would make a one-page list of all of my symptoms for my doctor and give it to the nurse. I included everything, even the things which did not seem significant to me, but were definitely not normal. I would keep a copy for myself during the appointment.

In most cases, the doctor would read the list and I wouldn't have to tell him every little thing freaking out in my body. Other doctors insisted I explain to them what I was feeling, so I would read my list to them. This list allowed me to detach from my symptoms so I could talk about them without getting upset, and it prevented me from forgetting things that may be important. I still use a list when I see the doctor. I make a note of any changes in my condition, any new treatments I've tried, and what I want from the doctor at our appointment. Whenever I meet a new doctor, I also make a point of telling the doctor about my spiritual practice and how it helps me from being overwhelmed by the constant pain and fatigue.

One doctor commented that I must be depressed because of the amount of pain and lack of sleep I experience daily. Since the sleep study proved my insomnia, he said either I was not really in that much pain, or I was in denial about my mental state. I had to explain to him once again about my Buddhist practice, and how I do not identify myself with the body. I asked him if he became depressed whenever his car broke down. He laughed, and seemed to understand my point.

If you cannot control your emotions when you visit your doctor, I recommend you make the time to visit a psychologist who is experienced with chronic pain patients to learn some tools to help you manage the effects your emotions. Even if you can control yourself most of the time, seeing a psychologist may still be beneficial because it will provide you a place to express everything you are going through. Chronic pain and fatigue are challenging conditions to treat, and they are exacerbated by lower mind states. The tools in this book may not be enough for everyone; most people living in pain need to talk out all of the difficult emotions that come with constant pain. With pain, there is frustration, loss, grief, and sometimes regret.

If you walk into your MD's office and start crying, he or she will want to fix the psychological component of your illness first. You may know the psychological difficulties you face are a result of the chronic pain and fatigue; unfortunately your doctor won't be certain. Clinical depression, in which there is an imbalance in the chemicals of the brain, can also cause pain and insomnia. Sometimes an antidepressant pill or psychotherapy works well enough to get the pain and fatigue under control so you can function. Other times the psychotherapy will merely help you gain control over your emotions so you can have an open discussion with your doctor about your physical symptoms.

No one else knows exactly what you experience.

I could share with you the vivid details of what I have endured through my illness, but you will never fully understand my experiences, just as I could never fully appreciate what you have been through. Each of us perceives events through a filter of conditioning we have developed over many, many years. So my perception of your experiences will be different from your actual experience. Even if you could somehow play them back for me on a movie screen, I cannot know what you have experienced, just as your perception of my life is different from what I actually experience.

Yet as humans, we have this burning desire to share our experiences, to be understood, and to be validated. The process of sharing experiences serves to bond humans to one another, and saves us from the deep-seated fear of being alone.

The truth is, you are alone, but only in your mind and experience as an individual. On a deeper – and permanent – level, we are One. We are eternal, infinite, pure, intelligent Light.

Take Action!

❖ Pay attention to how your thoughts change around different people and places.

❖ What thoughts are yours?

❖ Make a list of activities you can do and then invite a friend to join you to do one. If none of your friends are available, go by yourself. The next time you talk to your friend, tell them about your outing.

❖ Before your next doctor's appointment, make a list of everything you want to discuss. Include your symptoms, treatments, and what you want from the doctor.

A Little Secret About Stress

Stress is a warning to us. It occurs under one condition: when we are not doing what we know we should be doing at a particular moment. Stress indicates that immediate, deliberate and decisive action is required.

The world, including our bodies and mind, is constantly in flux. We have an amazing ability to instantly adapt to the changing environment within and without us. We experience stress when we resist making the adjustments necessary to bring our whole being into balance. Sometimes we resist physically through actions; other times we resist mentally by clinging to our ideas of the world and ourselves.

When we ignore the necessity for adaptation, our inner being, which knows exactly what we need to do at every single moment, pulls us one way while our thoughts and actions pull us in another. If we look at it closely, our mind under stress is like a rubber band stretched to its limit, as we try to go in two different directions. Stress is really that simple. It works in the same way as pain.

If you were to touch a hot stove, you would feel pain as your hand began to burn. When you lift something too heavy, you feel the strain of your muscles. The pain tells us to move our hand from the stove and put cold water on it. It tells us to not lift the object because it is too heavy. Pain is relatively easy to understand, and the body reacts quickly to it.

Stress, however, sometimes fools us. We rationalize why we may feel overwhelmed or anxious, and we continue doing what we are doing. We tell ourselves we must do this activity (or not do it) because it is socially correct or we want to please someone. Instead of recognizing the feelings of anxiety or frustration as symptoms of mental tension, we push the cause outside of ourselves; we decide the person or situation is the problem. The ego does not want to admit that it is both the source and the cure for stress.

It's unrealistic to think you should never feel angst. Humans are wonderfully imperfect; it is our imperfection that gives rise to creativity and innovation. If we were perfect, then there would be no need to explore new ways of doing or seeing things. Life would be boring and predictable. Stress is only a problem when you don't know what it is, when you forget it's your heart's way of telling you there is something else for you to do at this particular moment.

Our inner being, or heart, or soul, has access to everything all at once. It sees the world completely and more clearly than our rational mind ever could. It's the part of us that just "knows" what to do. We feel this part of us in the center of our chest, at our heart. Our inner being is our personal balance point in the ever-changing world and within our ever-changing bodies.

Whenever you feel stress, stop and examine exactly what you are doing, both physically and mentally. Many times when beginning a new project, we experience mental tension. This occurs because we jump ahead and see all the work in front of us, instead of focusing on the first task. Once we return our focus to the present task, stress disappears. Keep in mind the first task is often taking the time to create a plan for the project.

Stress can be paralyzing, as one overwhelming thought appears after another. It can emerge when you are sitting doing nothing. The secret is very simple, and worth repeating: stop and evaluate what you are doing, both physically and mentally. Ask your heart, what do I need to be doing, right now, at this moment? Then do it.

It's important to figure out what you *need* to be doing, not what you *think you should* be doing. The heart is demanding and not always logical. Your ego may tell you that you should stop at the store, but what you really need is to sit at the park or on the beach for a few minutes to rejuvenate in nature. If you ignore what your heart needs, at the store you will feel stress and have a very difficult time. Your heart will be pulling you towards the park, while your body and mind are pulling you towards the store, resulting in that profound mental tension. When you listen to what your heart needs, stress evaporates, leaving a very deep peace.

Take Action!

❖ Expand your mindfulness practice to watch for stress. When you encounter mental tension, deal with it immediately by stopping and asking yourself: what do I need to be doing right now? Then follow through by actually doing it.

❖ Be aware stress can occur when we get stuck in our plans. We may have the right list of things to do, but our inner being sometimes wants us to do them in a different order.

❖ In the beginning, your stress response may be very loud because it doesn't always get your attention. As you become more adept at listening to stress as a cue and following your heart, the stress response becomes more subtle. Instead of needing to be hit over the head with strong feelings of anxiety, a light tap on the shoulder with feelings of "something's not quite right" will suffice.

❖ As you pay attention, notice the times when physical pain turns into stress and vice-versa. To solve the mental tension, take care of both the mental and physical causes by doing what you need to with both your body and mind.

Personal Happiness &
Recreating Your Self Image

Most people assume if you are sick and/or in pain, you must be miserable. After all, every time they have had the flu or hurt themselves, they felt miserable, so you must too. Otherwise, you must not really be in severe pain...so they think.

What many people cannot conceive of is that the body can feel one way, and you, within your mind, can feel quite different. It doesn't mean the pain magically disappears. The body feels the pain, but the mind can focus so deeply on joy that the pain is miniscule in comparison. People who experience pain for short periods of time have no reason to learn how to do this. They feel miserable, in body and mind, and then the body heals and they go back to feeling good, in body and mind.

When the pain does not go away, and is not expected to go away, then you learn to "deal with it" as the doctors say. People learn to deal with pain in a variety of ways, and not all of them are beneficial. Some people embrace the misery and seek sympathy from everyone they meet. They expect special treatment, and when they don't get it, they believe the world is a cold, cruel place. Others sink into depression and isolate themselves from the world. They feel unworthy to participate in life because they are in pain. These are very dark places to live. There is an alternative: choosing joy over and over.

Personal happiness is not dependent upon external circumstances. Your body is an external circumstance. Happiness, true unconditional joy, deep inner peace, always exists within your heart. However, thoughts, attachments, and expectations get in the way of experiencing what is always there. In meditation, you'll begin to discover these ephemeral moments of perfect stillness. After practicing for a while, you may begin to notice the space in between the thoughts…that is where light and joy and peace are felt. All you have to do is quiet yourself enough to feel it. This is easy to say, but can be challenging to do. It gets easier with practice; and you only need to feel it once for a brief moment to know the truth of it. Let me repeat, personal happiness is not dependent upon external circumstances. Peace and joy exist right now, within you.

Every moment you have a choice: to experience peace or suffering. You can focus on your pain and wallow in the misery of it, the unfairness of it. Or, you can acknowledge your pain by acting within your physical limitations, and focus on the beauty of life. You say to your pain, "Yes, I know you are there, but right now I am going to watch a movie or read a book or listen to the birds chirp," and you focus on the feeling of gratitude for being able to do those things.

Over time, you will learn this new way of seeing yourself and your place in the world. It may not be what you expect or thought it would be. People may be confused by your happiness because they expect you to be miserable because you're in pain. That's OK. It's their problem, not yours. You can tell them, "I am happy today. It does not mean my body is better; it just means I am happy."

This process of living peacefully in joy requires you to recreate your self-image. You are not this fragile body. You are much more than simple flesh and blood. The more often you choose happiness despite what you may feel physically, the more apparent this will become to you.

Like many Americans, I wrapped my self-image into my career. I was a computer consultant. When I met someone and they asked me about myself, I told them I was a computer consultant. I did project management, software design and analysis, technical writing – I worked in all phases of software development. That was my life and I could talk about it for hours. It was who I was, and how I defined myself. When my illnesses progressed to the point where I could no longer work, I lost my life. I lost my personal definition of myself.

I became a sick, disabled woman. That's what the doctors told me, that's what my friends saw, and when I looked in the mirror I believed it. I forgot I was more than my fragile body. There was no one there to tell me otherwise. I fought against it as long as I could, but when I was forced to accept disability income, that solidified the new self-image. I hated it. I hated myself.

Fortunately my training as a Buddhist monk would not let me go so easily. I continued to meditate, even though I couldn't sit up on my own. I had to lean against the wall or use pillows to prop myself up in bed while I focused on the Light my Teacher had shown me over and over. It was sometimes tortuous, but my spirit would not let me stop. Even completely exhausted, something within me each day would not let me rest until I at least tried to meditate.

I had promised my Teacher I would share what he had given me, so I poured every ounce of energy I could access into teaching anyone who wanted to learn about meditation. With my students, I relearned all of the basics of meditation and mindfulness practice. In those moments, meditating with my students, I no longer felt my body. All that existed was joy and pure light.

Slowly, a new self-image emerged. I became a meditation teacher. And when I published the book I wrote before the illness, I became an author. (My first published book is *Worlds of Power, Worlds of Light*.) The old self continued to push forward, as I had to visit doctor after doctor for treatments for the body, and meet with lawyers to fight for SSDI benefits. However, with every class I taught and every time I sat down to meditate, I remembered: I am one of Buddha's monks. Remembering this allowed me to let go of the image of the sick, disabled woman. As I let go, a new self grew all by itself.

We don't always know what the new self will be like; Eternity takes care of it for us. I had no idea what a Buddhist monk in San Diego was like, or what a meditation teacher should be like. My Teacher ordained me as a monk, but did not leave behind a monastery to help me. I had my Teacher as a model, but I am not him. It would not have worked if I tried to copy him; I had to let go and jump in without knowing exactly how one is supposed to be a meditation teacher and monk.

Many people who experience chronic pain or illness pass through what Elizabeth Kübler Ross described as the Five Stages of Grief. She wrote about the loss of life; however, even if your chronic pain is not from a terminal illness, you still experience a type of death when pain changes your life. You may experience some or all of these stages during your personal journey. In her book, she described them as: Denial, Anger, Bargaining, Depression, and Acceptance. I suggest there be one more stage added: Rebirth. While acceptance of your condition is crucial, creating a new life for yourself is equally important. The rebirth allows you to discover all of the possibilities waiting for you, no matter if your body has six months or sixty years left on this earth.

When you decide you are ready to have a new self-image, all you need to do is let go of the image you have now and go exploring. Try new things. Make a list of things that excite or interest you. Perhaps you've always wanted to learn a new language. Take a class at your local community college or purchase a book or CD you can use at home. Or maybe you would like to paint; go buy some canvas, some brushes and some paint. Then play. No matter how silly or how unlike you it is, if it sounds interesting, check it out. You may be very surprised.

You may not be able to do things the way others have done them. Don't let this stop you. Experiment until you find a way to do it in a way that works for you. Look at the projects you want to accomplish, and break them into tiny pieces. It's taken me years to write this book because I couldn't sit down to write for hours and hours. I had to write for a few minutes, then stop and rest, and then write for a few more minutes. Over time, drop by drop, the pages were filled. The same is true for all of the projects I do. Of course I would like to do things faster; however my body is slow. Knowing this helps me to remember to spend time on only the things I love.

Keep exploring, and allow your self-image to continue to change. When you meet new people, instead of saying you are disabled, you can tell them you are a painter or you love to watch movies or read science fiction or whatever it is you are playing with now. If they know about your chronic pain and ask you about it, mention a few words and then change the subject back to the fun things in your life. And of course, ask them about the fun things in their lives too!

 Take Action!

❖ Allow yourself to dream…forget about all of your limitations, both physical and financial…dream of what you would like to do or be.

❖ Make a list of dreams, then sort through them and see if you can manifest one or two of them in some way that fits your current circumstances. Have fun with it, and don't hold onto any expectations of how it should or should not be.

❖ Try at least one new activity each month or each season.

Impeccability

Out of denial about the sickness that holds
My body hostage, I realize my Ignorance
And can now begin the journey to health
And learn the Truth of Healing.
Separating emotional baggage from physical issues
Is part of the process
Sorting it all out, and dealing with each piece
One day at a time,
One meal at a time.
Learning to let myself rest, relax, recuperate.

So deeply in love with Jim.
Ready to share everything:
The joy, the fear, the bliss, the excitement of life.
I want to live
Actively, healthy, brightly.
I must accept where I am, who I am, what I am
In order to move past the limitations.
How can you grow past your limits
if you don't know what they are?

There is time for it all.
Bird song at sunset
Parrot calls laced through a melody of chirps
The ocean tide turns
I am here now
And ready to be Free.

Impeccability means to always do your best and expand your limits. In order to do this, you first must learn where your limits are. Then, you take one baby step past them. Most likely, you will fall on your face, which is always fine because you've done your best. So you get up, dust yourself off, and you try again. Fall down, get up – it is one step. Eventually, you will succeed. In that tiny success, you have expanded your limits. When you're ready, you repeat the process. Always remember: Fall down, get up – it's one step.

How you decide to push your limits is entirely up to you. Perhaps you would like to cook a special meal without help. For this example, part of the exercise would be to select food packages you can open on your own. (I have trouble opening jars, so for me bottled pasta sauce would not be a good choice.) Your meal option would be just beyond your comfort level. If it's way too complicated or time consuming, you'll frustrate yourself. My mother has a wonderful recipe for pecan cinnamon rolls made from scratch; however it's an all-day project, which is way beyond my reach right now. Prepare yourself for the task and know exactly what you're getting yourself into. It may sound like a simple thing for someone else, but we're talking about your limits, not theirs. Remember, we grow in baby steps.

Maybe cooking doesn't interest you. Instead you might be more interested in improving your body's functionality, range of motion, and endurance. An exercise program will allow you to do this, provided you approach it in an impeccable way.

I decided to learn Tai Chi for this purpose. I've

always loved martial arts, however I knew my body could no longer tolerate being punched in a Karate class or being thrown around in an Aikido class. My Teacher had recommended Tai Chi to me many years ago, so I finally decided to follow his suggestion.

My first attempt at learning Tai Chi resulted in total failure. I found a neighborhood dojo and joined the weekly class. The teacher was excellent; however the class was geared for healthy people and at the time my illness was completely out of control. I forced myself to remain on my feet during the entire class. The pain and fatigue escalated and caused my mind to shut down. I was unable to learn anything, even when the teacher worked with me one-on-one at the end of class. Simply driving home after class took all of my willpower. Within a couple of months, my doctor insisted I stop.

After taking the time to gain some control over my pain levels and learning to pace myself, I tried again. This time I found a senior citizen Tai Chi class more appropriate to my level. Of course at first I tried to do too much. I thought surely I could keep up with a group of 70 and 80 year old people. I was wrong. I forgot to be impeccable; I compared myself to them, instead of comparing myself to my prior self and pushing my own limits.

Fortunately, I did remember to get up after falling down. I re-examined my goals: I wanted to learn the short form of Tai Chi. I gave up trying to do the 30-minutes of warm up Qi-Gong exercises. Instead, when I arrived for class, I would rest from driving and do a few of my own stretches to warm up my body in the way it needed. When we practiced the Short Form, I would watch my pain level carefully and sit down as soon as it began to rise, and then get up as soon as it returned to normal. I made an effort to learn only one small part of the form each week, and then practiced at home up to the point in the sequence I had learned.

Sometimes it took me two weeks to learn one move. In the case of the Four Corners, it took me five weeks to learn, because I tried to learn the entire thing at once. I had to ask the teacher to show me only one corner, and then stop him before he went on to the next. Even though each corner was the same, my mind could only absorb one small section at a time. After a year, I was able to do the 18 move Short Form on my own. My form could be much better, so I continue to practice and make improvements every week. Over the course of this time, I have grown stronger, both physically and mentally.

Don't confuse impeccability with perfection. People want a perfectly manicured landscape, or a perfectly clean home, or a perfectly healthy body. Perfection is a state of mind. What you consider perfect may not be what someone else considers perfect. Also, your idea of perfection is transitory. What was perfect yesterday has flaws today. The object did not change; your perception of it did. Your big accomplishment last week was perfect then; today you see all the ways it could have been better.

Celebrate all of your accomplishments, both big and small. Use them to inspire you to keep growing. Beware of perfectionism sneaking in to rob you of your glory. When you are honest with yourself, you know what you are capable of doing and when you are ready to push beyond those capabilities. Accept that you will fall down in the process; simply get up and keep moving forward. To live impeccably means to always do your best, and then push yourself a tiny bit further.

 Take Action!

❖ Take stock of all of your limitations and your current level of ability.

❖ Select a single area of your life you would like to improve, and begin the practice of impeccability today.

❖ When you are ready, address other areas of your life. Do everything in baby steps.

❖ Apply impeccability to your meditation practice every day.

Goals And Having
A Purpose For Being

Long, crisp nights –
Twilight comes so early,
And then suddenly,
Winter Solstice is upon us.
The power shifts to
Expansion
Longer days filled with Light.
A time to begin anew.
Take stock of who you are
Today – not who you were yesterday.
What dreams are you dreaming for yourself?

Goals are a wonderful way to focus your energy and attention. Some people have modest goals, like to read a book. Other people have more grandiose goals, like becoming President of the United States. Whatever your goal is, to accomplish it you will need to invest time and energy into it.

There is a great deal of power in choosing your own goals. Many people don't embrace this power; instead others push them around. Perhaps you had an idea to do something, and someone close to you shot the idea down. This person told you all the things that could go wrong and that it was a waste of time. Maybe they said it would be too hard. So you took this person's suggestion of how to spend your time instead of pursuing your idea. I don't believe most people do this maliciously. I think they are merely trying to protect the ones they love. And sometimes, we do this to ourselves.

When you live in chronic pain, your time and energy are more limited than other people. That doesn't mean you cannot have goals. Rather, it means you will want to select your goals carefully. If you have only one dollar to spend, you'd want to spend it on something you really want instead of wasting it on junk, right?

We all have our lists of "want to's" and "have to's" in our lives. Sometimes they line up, where something we want and have to do are one in the same, and sometimes they don't. Making your "want to" list a priority in your life will keep you motivated to do all the "have to" things. Perhaps you have many doctor appointments that you have to keep. In this case, build some fun time into your schedule by making an appointment for yourself to do something fun from your "want to" list.

Combining the "want to" and "have to" lists is a valuable option. I have to rest often. I've always been an active person, so resting is one of my least favorite things to do. If it's my body that needs rest, and not my mind, I watch a video. Watching movies and my favorite shows falls under my "want to" list, so combining it with my rest time makes it easier to take care of myself.

Invest the time to sit down and consider what you want to do with your time and energy. Many times when we are engulfed by chronic pain, it feels like we can do nothing. Life becomes a series of doctor appointments and tests, followed by the disappointing news that there's nothing the doctor can do to alleviate the pain. While it's important to keep checking with your doctor – there are new discoveries in medicine everyday – it's also important for you to make time for the things you love. And if you don't know what you love, then discovering it is your first goal.

If you enjoy going to museums, then schedule a day for you to go. Don't try to squeeze it in around the other things in your life; instead make the museum trip your activity for the entire day. You may only go for an hour, and then need to go home and rest. However, as you're sitting at home resting, your mind will be filled with all the wonderful things you saw while you were out. And knowing you achieved your goal of visiting the museum will give you the motivation to work towards your next one.

Writing down your goals is an essential step. When you put something on paper, it makes it more tangible. After you see the words spelled out, you may discover you liked the idea of the goal more than the goal itself. If this is the case, cross that one out and look inside for what truly interests you. Don't let yourself dismiss something just because it sounds difficult or even impossible.

Perhaps you would like to see the inside of the Grand Canyon, however there's no way you could hike for eight hours or sit on the back of a mule for four hours. Instead of giving up on your dream, you could make a long-term plan to save up money for a helicopter tour of the Grand Canyon instead. While it's not exactly the same, it is close.

Dream big and then be creative about how to

accomplish your goals. Because you live with chronic pain, you will need to do things differently than other people. Try to make time every week to work towards your goals. If you miss a week don't feel bad, just pick up where you left off as soon as you are able.

Update your goal list every month or every quarter. As we grow, our goals change. Something that seemed very important to you last month may not be as interesting next month. Now don't change it just because it became difficult. You have to expect challenges and opposition – that comes with any endeavor, whether you have a healthy body or not.

Your goals, large or small, give you a reason to get up in the morning. Goals point you in a specific direction, allowing you to efficiently use your time and energy. They make your life exciting and give you something to share with your loved ones. When you reach one goal, enjoy the fleeting sense of satisfaction and then quickly move on to the next one.

Celebrate your successes and learn from your failures. You have nothing to prove; goals are for the pure delight of working towards something that is important to you. There is as much joy in the journey to the goal as there is in its achievement.

We have the ability to create a sense of meaning in our own lives, and goals are one way to do this. There is a great deal of power in setting and meeting goals, especially ones of our own choosing. Take hold of this power today and create your own path in the world.

Take Action!

❖ Make a list of your "have to's" and "want to's" on two separate pieces of paper.

❖ Are there any activities you can combine from the two lists?

❖ Make a list of dream goals – allow yourself the freedom to write whatever you want, without regard to what is possible or feasible. Forget about what others may or may not say; this list is for you alone.

❖ Pick one goal from your list that you can accomplish. Then break it down into very small pieces and work on one piece each week.

❖ Every morning have a plan of what you will do for the day. If you need rest, you may decide to watch a movie or take a nap. If you have some energy, perhaps you'll spend an hour on a project. Stay flexible and change when needed, but choose what to do every day. As *The I Ching* points out: "It furthers one to have some place to go."

Taking Care Of The Body

The body is a temple.
You do not worship the temple.
You worship God inside the temple.
Take care of your temple, your body,
So you have an inviting place to worship.

Pacing

When I was first taught the concept of Pacing, I did not believe it could help me. I was too busy; I had too many things I wanted to do to slow down. I also knew from experience if I stopped to rest, then I wouldn't be able to get up again, sometimes for days at a time. In short, I was very stubborn and impatient.

Pacing allows you, over time, to build up your endurance. The theory is as follows: If you rest the body at the first sign of increased pain, and stay resting until the pain recedes back to your normal level, you will have more "up" time and less "down" time.

When I was first introduced to this concept, my pain was completely out of control. Every task I accomplished was by sheer willpower. Once I got myself moving, I built up a degree of momentum and could keep going – physically. Mentally, my mind would shut down into what others have termed "fibrofog" and I would forget what I was doing in the middle of doing it. Not a good state to be in while driving! Eventually, my muscles would revolt by not responding, causing me to fall down and forcing me to stop dead in my tracks at the most inconvenient times.

The psychologist who ran the pain support group I attended suggested I pick one thing each day, and make accomplishing it enough for me to feel productive. Once I finished my one task, I would let myself rest for however long my body wanted to, even if it was all day. Only if I felt rested, would I allow myself to do a second activity.

In the beginning, my one task was taking a shower. Washing my long hair increased the pain in my shoulders, arms and hands, so I would always have to rest anyway. (I never counted meditation as a task because for me it's like eating or breathing; meditation is not an optional thing I could skip for a day like showering.) Every morning, I would wake up slowly, eat breakfast and meditate, and when I was ready, I took a shower. Then I would rest until the pain diminished some. I would complete the process by drying my hair and getting dressed. Once I was dressed, I let myself rest for the remainder of the day. At first, it took me until the afternoon to make it into the shower. Some days I was not able to dry my hair, and wound up back in my pajamas in bed.

A big mistake I made kept me from progressing. I thought reading on the couch counted as resting. It doesn't. Reading uses your mind, your arms, and your hands. Even if you have something to hold the book open for you, you still have to lift your hand every few minutes to turn the page. I had to have someone in the support group point this out to me when I complained the pacing wasn't working.

I tried to sleep as much as possible, but when the pain is screaming at you, sleep doesn't come easily. Most shows on daytime television are boring repeats (in my opinion), so I learned to record the few shows I did enjoy. That way I could rest whenever I needed to, instead of on the television's schedule, and I didn't have to subject myself to the commercials. Lying with my body fully supported, and my mind engaged in a television show or movie was the only way I could get myself to rest. Over the course of time, I also discovered audio books and lectures on CDs that would keep me resting and entertained while I listened to them with my portable CD or MP3 player.

You have probably already figured out that boredom is one of the worst places to be when in chronic pain. Lying there thinking of all the things you could or should be doing is a form of torture. Boredom leads to immense frustration and suffering because you know your body cannot go out to find entertainment. It's crucial to find videos or CDs you enjoy to keep your mind occupied while you let your entire body rest.

If your chronic pain is out of control – where the pain is unbearable all of the time – then I recommend starting where I did, with one task each day. It doesn't have to be the same task every day, but the tasks should take about the same amount of energy. Maybe on one day you shower, and the next you wash dishes, fold laundry, or some other type of light housework. After several weeks, you'll begin to notice the fluctuations in your pain levels before the task, after the task, and after resting. Give yourself at least two weeks or a month before adding a second task to your day.

When you're ready to add more to your day, move on to the second task *after* you have rested and recovered from the first. Pick something that can wait if your pain levels start to rise. For example, if you fold laundry and your arms start to hurt, immediately stop and rest. Once the pain has receded, then start folding laundry again. A trick I use is to fold laundry while watching television; I'll fold clothes during the commercials, and once the show comes back on, I stop and rest. I also began my practice of Tai Chi the same way – during commercials I would do the movements I learned in class, and then rest during the program.

Make pacing part of your mindfulness practice; be aware of the rising pain levels and deal with it immediately by resting. When your car gets low on gas, you go the gas station and fill it up, no big deal. Pacing is very similar; when your body starts to feel pain, you rest until it recedes, no big deal. You wouldn't drive your car until it completely runs out of gas, so why push your body until it's empty of energy?

Pacing does work. In the beginning, I had an average of about 15 minutes per day of active "up" time. Over the course of a few months, I was able to have multiple 15-minute sessions of "up" time each day. After several more months, I was able to begin combining my sessions into 30-minutes of "up" time each day. Over a few years, I increased it again to a consistent hour of activity each day. (Of course, I had the tendency to blow my progress by over-doing it and have a setback.) Now I'm up to 2 to 3 hours of activity on most days. Sometimes I still do too much, and suffer the consequences of being laid out for a few days. This is an ongoing learning process, especially with an illness where pain levels can skyrocket for no apparent reason.

I strongly encourage you to practice pacing by making it part of your daily life. For me, it helps to think of my body like a vehicle, which removes the emotional turmoil. If my body doesn't have the strength to do something, then I find another way. If it's tired, I let it rest and recharge. There's no need to abuse the body because it doesn't work like other people's bodies or because it doesn't work like it used to. Your body is the way it is today, and the best option is to learn how to drive it appropriately to get optimum performance.

It will take you longer to do the things most people do in a few minutes. You are not most people; your energy is being drained by pain, and the more pain your body experiences, the faster the drain.

You may want to explain to your friends and family about pacing so you will get the support you need. Be sure to communicate with them when you need to rest, and then follow through by actually stopping and resting. (If you say, "I need to rest" and then you keep going, they won't believe you the next time. It's the "Little Boy Who Cried Wolf" all over again.) There was a time when I sat down on a sidewalk in New York City because I needed to rest. I was too tired to care where I sat. My friend was a little embarrassed, but after that, she knew I meant it when I said I needed to rest.

You are the only one who knows what your body can handle at any particular moment, so it's important to communicate your needs to the people you are with. It's even more important to be honest with yourself.

Pacing practice begins with watching your pain levels. Take a full day to rest so you can get an accurate read on what your normal pain levels are. During this day, write down your pain level, using a scale from 0 (no pain) to 10 (extreme, unbearable pain). At the end of the day, review the numbers and remember what your "normal" pain level is.

Beginning the next day as you do any activity, no matter how minor or mundane, watch your pain levels. If the pain increases, then stop immediately and rest until the pain recedes to your typical level. Then start the activity again. Look for different ways of doing activities so they don't put as much strain on your body. Allow yourself to rest as often as necessary. Gradually, you will be able to stay active for longer periods of time.

Take Action!

❖ What is your pain level right now, on a scale of 0 to 10, where 0 = no pain and 10 = excruciating, can't stand up without help?

❖ Is that your average pain level?

❖ What activities increase your pain? Can you do them differently? If not, is there someone you can ask or hire to do them for you?

❖ Suggestions for Household Maintenance and Pacing:

o Empty the dishwasher slowly. If lifting three plates at a time increases your pain, put them away one at a time instead.

o Put the most often used dishes and glasses on the lowest shelves.

o If you cannot afford to pay a cleaning service company, spread the cleaning chores for each area over several days. In the bathroom, clean the sink and mirror on the first day, scrub the toilet on the second, scrub the tub on the third, and wash the floor on the fourth. During the following week, do the kitchen one section per day. Then the week after that, dust and vacuum one room each day. Ten to twenty minutes of cleaning a few days each week will cause less pain than trying to clean for three hours in a single day.

Body Rhythms:
Time To Eat, Time To Sleep

The earth has its own rhythms: the seasons of the year, day and night, and the rising and receding of the ocean's tides. Each season and time of day is conducive to certain activities more so than others. If you want to visit the tide pools along the coast, you must do so at low tide or there won't be much to see.

Just like the earth, our bodies have a rhythm of their own. We can discover this rhythm and fine-tune our activities to make the most of our body's capabilities. Through mindfulness, we pay attention to the needs of the body. In turn, the body pays attention to what we do in order to anticipate the resources it has available.

When we live with chronic pain, our energy is sapped. We may not feel hungry, or we may feel we simply don't have the energy to eat, so we skip meals. The body responds to the lack of food, and to irregular eating patterns, by conserving even more energy for vital functions, like breathing and pumping blood. When it does get food, it devours it and hoards the energy from it like a starving beggar.

We can support the body by feeding it at roughly the same time each day. The meals do not need to be large or sophisticated; just a small amount of nutrition at predictable intervals will allow the body to find its rhythm.

Some people find it easier on their digestion to eat five to six tiny meals each day, so they are eating every two to three hours. For me, eating three meals and a small snack between lunch and dinner works best for my body.

By giving my body food at regular times each day - within an hour or two of getting up in the morning, mid-day, late afternoon, and evening – my body knows it will get the fuel it needs to sustain both the vital functions and the activities I do. Even just a small bowl of rice or cereal or salad or piece of toast is enough to keep the body's trust that it will be given the food it needs.

Look at when and how often you eat and see if you can find the pattern. If there is no pattern, then take the time to develop an eating habit. Of course, you'll want to include healthy, nutritious food, and we'll talk more about nutrition later, but for now, we're more concerned with creating a schedule. It may take several weeks or months to discover your personal rhythm when it comes to food.

Start by figuring out how soon after waking your body wants to eat. Some people need food right away; others need to move around first, so they shower or exercise first. A few may prefer to stretch and meditate before eating the first meal of the day. This is a process of discovering what works best for your body.

Once you've figured out when your breakfast time is, then use mindfulness to learn when you need to fill up again. Many times I don't feel hungry; rather I'll begin to notice an increase in fatigue or even pain. Most people don't associate hunger with fatigue. When you're tired, you want to rest and not eat. But once I learned that was my body's way of telling me it needed more fuel, I figured out how long I could go between breakfast and lunch. By eating a light lunch before the fatigue hits me, I can eat and take a short rest before continuing with my day's activities. Again, we experiment to find what works.

Because of the medication and the inability to do vigorous exercise, I gained some weight. This made me not want to snack in between meals. What I soon discovered though, is by dinner time I would be too exhausted to cook. Once I added a 4 o'clock snack to my daily eating schedule, I was able to make dinner without feeling like I was about to pass out.

Throughout the day, watch your body and mind to learn what the best times are to re-fuel your system. Then stick with that rhythm, even if it means putting a granola bar in your pocket when you go out so you can eat on your body's time.

The other part of the body's rhythm is sleep. Most of us with chronic pain have a great deal of difficulty sleeping. Just like with eating, if we don't give the body regular rest periods, it will conserve energy for vital functions. Then it will conk out whenever it has a chance. This leaves us feeling too exhausted to undertake anything, because we don't know if we'll have the energy to actually do it.

For at least a full month, go to bed at the same time each night, and get up at the same time each morning. Then adjust the times earlier or later as needed. If your situation is such that you have to get up at a certain time on most days, then you'll have only your bedtime to adjust. On the days you don't have to get up, make yourself get up close to the regular time.

By spending the same amount of time in bed each night, your body will begin to learn how long it has to rest. If you spend an extra two or three hours in bed on the weekends, the body will be confused and feel deprived when you force it up earlier. During the day, you can always take a short nap if you need it. However, give your body a set amount of time at night.

The time you spend in bed at night is a rest period. The body may or may not actually sleep. For many of us, we will toss and turn for most of the night. Instead of fighting to sleep, we can use the allotted time to rest and relax. If sleep comes, we enjoy it; if not, we still allow the body to rest as much as it can.

Where we sleep is important. The bed is a sanctuary, and should be used for only sleep and sex. When we sit on the bed to talk on the phone, fold laundry, watch tv, or do other activities, we miss the opportunity to teach our body that the bed is for rest and relaxation. Just like the body can learn when it's time to quiet and meditate by sitting in the same spot each day, the body learns when it's time to sleep by using our bed only for rest.

Many of us like to read before bed; however consider the type of book you are reading in bed – does it help create a sense of rest and relaxation? If it's an exciting thriller, then that book might be better on the couch. Observe your sleep after reading, and then decide if that book is conducive to rest or not.

At night, take a look around your bedroom. Is it dark and quiet? Many electronics have small lights that can be very bright when the rest of the room is dark.

Light wakes us up. It can be helpful to cover up those little lights, as well as invest in dark shades to cover the windows. If noise is an issue, you can muffle the sounds by playing a CD with relaxing ocean sounds or white noise.

Temperature and humidity can also be a factor that affects sleep quality. Most people prefer it to be cool; however you'll need to discover what is comfortable to you. If your nose feels dry, adding a humidifier can make a huge difference. On the other hand, if it's stuffy, you can try a de-humidifier.

A nightly ritual can help prepare us for the evening's rest. Drinking a small glass of water, washing our face, brushing our teeth and hair, spending a minute or two smiling at ourselves in the mirror, are all opportunities to let go of the day's worries and sink into relaxation. We can use the rituals to help us look forward to relaxing in bed. When we climb under the covers, we can close our eyes, take a deep breath, and let go.

In the morning, when it's time to rise, allow yourself to stretch and slowly bring your body back into a state of activity. Smiling before getting out of bed is always a great way to start the day.

Life rarely goes according to plan, so there is no doubt your eating and sleeping rhythms will be interrupted. When this happens, acknowledge the change in resources. Be extra gentle with your body for the next several days as you return to your normal schedule. When we miss a meal or our rest time is shortened, it may take a day or two before we feel it. By then, we may have forgotten about the missed meal or the late night. We can accommodate the interruption by planning our activities for the next few days with flexibility. If you feel unusually tired or grumpy, remember why, and be good to your body. Instead of running a bunch of errands, you may need to catch up on the movies you've been waiting to watch.

The body is a creature of habit. It loves routines because they make it easier for the entire system to manage its resources. By paying attention to the needs of our body, it will learn to trust that it will get the fuel and rest it requires to function at its best.

Take Action!

❖ Listen to your body first thing in the morning. Does it want food right away? Or would it prefer to wait a short time. If you don't normally eat breakfast, try giving your body something light about an hour after you wake up. Eat at the same time each day for a week or two, and then adjust as necessary. Keep experimenting until you find a schedule that makes your body happy.

❖ Go to bed and get up in the morning at the same time each day. Allow your body to learn when it's time to rest. If you feel exhausted in the morning, try going to bed earlier or getting up later. After a month or two, you will begin to automatically wake at the same time each day. Reinforce this habit by actually getting out of bed when you wake up.

❖ During the day, allow yourself to take a short nap if you need it. Pay attention to what time of day you take the nap, and if it affects your ability to rest at night. If it does, try taking a nap earlier in the day next time.

❖ When you are in bed, it is a time of rest and relaxation. Know that you may or may not fall asleep. Simply allow the body to rest and relax.

❖ Honor your body's routine of eating and sleeping. If you do need to disrupt them, then get back on track as soon as possible.

Decisions About Disability Income

When your body has difficulty performing the activities of daily living, you are disabled. The label of "disabled" is a difficult one to accept because it pulls apart our definition of self. The degree of disability varies widely among different people, and for some of us, it varies from day to day. Whether the disability is mild or severe, it can help to step back and realize we are much more than the body.

To interact with others and explore the world, we use our bodies. So their level of functioning has a powerful impact on how we participate in life. Ignoring our impairments prevents us from making the most of what functioning we do have, and often leads us to abusing the body and weakening it further.

If you discover you are having trouble performing daily activities such as eating, cleaning, playing, and working, then it's time to do an honest assessment. The first step is to learn your problem areas and seek out ways to accommodate the needs of your body. This may mean doing the activity differently, taking frequent rest breaks, or changing to another activity altogether.

The American Disability Act requires employers to make reasonable accommodations for employees who are disabled. This requirement is intentionally vague, so it fits the needs of a wide variety of individuals and employers.

A company must function in order to stay in business, so it's important to carefully consider what a reasonable accommodation is for each situation. A bank teller taking a 10-minute rest break every hour probably would not be reasonable, because customers cannot be left waiting. However, a chair for the bank teller to sit in so he does not have to stand all day is reasonable. A data-entry clerk requesting a rest break every hour in a business where she could stay late to make up the time is a reasonable request. As you can imagine, there is a limit to what accommodations can be made in the workplace.

If you are disabled and in need of accommodation, it is important to first discuss the issue with your doctor. He or she may not be aware of how much your pain and/or illness are affecting you. Dropping things, not being able to lift as much weight as you used to, and needing to rest frequently are important symptoms to share with your doctor.

To prepare for your visit, think about your day in terms of daily functioning. Consider what you cannot do, or what you need to do special, and make a note of these things. Ask your doctor to help you come up with a plan to make the necessary accommodations. When you have special needs in the workplace, it's always a good idea to obtain a note from your doctor outlining these. You may not need it, but it can provide the proof some employers need in order to take your request seriously.

When you approach your manager or human resource director, try to see the situation from both sides. You want to work, and they want to make sure the work is done correctly and on time. Keep this goal in mind and approach it as a discussion. Be prepared to offer your solution, and be open to other ideas as well.

Sometimes the disability becomes so severe that we can no longer work. This can be devastating both emotionally and financially. Many of us tie our identity to our work, so when we lose our job, we lose ourselves. This is a real loss, and we go through a grieving process as a new identity emerges. By being conscious of what is happening, we can move through the suffering and discover a whole new self.

In this situation, we are faced with the decision about disability income. It's important to remember this is a decision to be made based on logic and not emotion. Most of us put a high value on work, and accepting disability income can make us feel less valuable as a human being.

We may find ourselves hiding our physical difficulties from others or making excuses such as, "I just didn't sleep well last night, I'll be better tomorrow." This emotional response can deter us from applying for disability, prevent us from getting the support we need, and cause us to give up if our claim is denied.

When we sit down with our doctors and perform a functional analysis of our body, it has no bearing on our worth as a human being. While there will certainly be an emotional upheaval, it's important to stay focused on the issue of disability. Doctors do not like to admit their patient is disabled. For the doctor, it must feel like a failure to say in writing they cannot fix the patient. For the patient, this feeling of hopelessness is even stronger. Still the issue remains a logical one: either the body can perform or it cannot.

At this time of transition, a psychologist can be a

valuable ally. This specialist can help us process and deal with the loss, and they can note any mental or cognitive issues that play a part in our disability.

Whether your employer offers disability insurance or if you are applying for federal disability insurance (SSDI), proper documentation is essential. Unfortunately, your word and the statements by your loved ones are not enough. Your disability must be clearly noted in your medical records by your doctors.

Obtain a copy of your medical records and read the doctor's notes. When reviewing a claim, insurance adjusters look for signs, not symptoms. A symptom is something the patient tells the doctor, such as: "The patient reports widespread pain." A sign is the result of a test or exam, such as: "A tender point exam reveals 18 out of 18 tender points." The signs noted by your doctors will support the diagnosis they make for your condition.

If you have insurance either on your own or through an employer, read the policy carefully. Some policies have limits on mental disabilities. In this case if you have a disability that affects your body, it's important your doctor records in your medical chart that you have a physical condition causing your disability. Insurance companies are in the business of making money, and they will attempt to not pay a policy if legally possible.

While rare, I have heard of a case where an employer encouraged a woman to quit when she became ill, instead of having her file for the company's disability insurance. Because of the emotional turmoil she felt at not being able to work, she gave in and quit. It can be challenging when you don't feel well, but it's to your benefit to know and stand up for your rights.

If you work and pay taxes, you are paying for disability insurance, called SSDI. To be eligible to collect, you must pay into the system for a certain amount of time, which varies based on age.

This federal insurance is available for people who have been or are expected to be disabled for at least 12 months. The clock begins after your last day of work. Most people will need to wait the full 12 months before they can apply. Some states have short-term disability insurance; you can check with your state's government to see if this is available.

To collect disability insurance, you must be "totally" disabled, which means you cannot work at your current job or at any other type of substantial gainful employment. Basically, you cannot work and support yourself because your body or mental state prevents you from doing so. It does *not* mean you are bed-ridden. You may still be able to cook a meal, wash dishes, and go to the grocery store. Their definition of "total disability" simply means you cannot consistently work at a place of employment. If you have limited assets, you may qualify for the federal SSI program, even if you are not eligible for SSDI.

The process of filing a disability insurance claim can be time consuming and confusing. There are many lawyers willing to help; however they will take a portion of your payments. In most cases, you may want to begin the process with your doctor and consult a lawyer only if you are denied. However, every case is different, so you'll need to determine if your situation requires legal advice.

For the two federal programs, SSDI and SSI, you

can learn the rules and requirements by reviewing the official government website: www.ssa.gov/disability or you can call Social Security at 1-800-772-1213 for an appointment to discuss your case. Keep in mind if you call, the operator cannot give you legal or medical advice.

Many SSDI claims are denied, and will require you to request a review. There is a list of conditions for which claims are automatically approved, provided all required documentation is included in your medical records. You can find this list on the SSA's website.

If your claim is denied, you may want to consider hiring a lawyer. For SSDI cases, there is a fixed limit on the amount a lawyer can charge, and they cannot charge you anything if your claim is not approved. For SSDI, there is the initial application phase; if you are denied, you file a written appeal. If that is denied, then you can request a judicial review in front of a local judge. At this point, it's very helpful to have a lawyer who can ask you the right questions to help the judge understand your case. If the judge denies your claim, there is another appeal option in front of a Federal judge.

Because the process takes so long, people who are approved typically receive a large check for retroactive benefits. If you decide to hire a lawyer, take your time interviewing several candidates and select the one with whom you feel most comfortable.

Once your disability claim is approved, continue to check in with your doctor at least once a year. Update your doctor on your current functional status and discuss any new treatment options. SSDI and insurance companies routinely review active claims, so it's important they can access medical records from a doctor you trust.

SSDI or your private insurance company will also send you forms to fill out periodically. Be sure to complete these accurately and keep a copy for your records. You may want to mail them with signature confirmation to know they were delivered on time.

Along with financial support, SSDI recipients also become eligible for Medicare. The Medicare program varies by state, and you can learn what options are available to you through www.Medicare.gov by following the prompts to enter your zip code. If you want to purchase a Medicare supplement plan, you must do so within the first six months of beginning Medicare. After six months, insurance companies have the right to do an underwriting process and if you're disabled, it's unlikely you will be accepted. Once you become eligible for Medicare, take the time to review your health insurance options carefully.

If your condition improves and you want to try working, the Social Security Administration (SSA, which runs SSDI and SSI) has implemented several programs to make it easier to explore working without losing your benefits.

Communicating with SSA is essential throughout the process. If you call to tell them you are going to try working, and never call them back, they will assume you are no longer disabled and will want to collect any money they sent you after the nine month trial work period. If you try working and find you cannot, be sure to report this to the SSA in writing.

Each year the program details may change, so it's important to review www.ssa.gov/disability for the most up-to-date information. Currently, there is a trial work period that lasts 60 months, during which your benefits will not be affected. During this 60-month period if you are able to earn a certain amount or work 80 hours during a month, it counts towards a nine-month goal. Once you have accumulated nine months within a rolling 60-month period, then your benefits are affected.

After the trial work period, your benefits will not be paid during the future months in which your earnings were "substantial." As of this writing, substantial means $1070 per month. You may deduct any expenses incurred because of your disability, such has having to take a taxi instead of public transportation. This period then lasts 36 months. If during this time you find you cannot work because of your disability, your benefits are immediately reinstated without having to wait for an approval.

However, during the entire process it is crucial that you communicate with SSA about your progress. If you discover you cannot work, you will still need to fill out the appropriate forms and your doctor will need to send your medical records.

In addition to the time period and income guidelines, the SSA also offers vocational training and an employment network to help people who want to try working. You can visit www.ssa.gov/work for the latest information.

Living with a disability, whether it is mild or severe, is a daily challenge. Not only are we confronted by society's view of what it means to be disabled, we also must deal with our own conditioning. For most of us, admitting we are disabled is a brutal blow to our sense of self. However, once we begin to realize we are much more than a body, we discover we have much to offer the world.

While we may not be able to translate our unique gifts into a paying career, we can still explore and share what we love with those around us. In doing so, we become a productive and active member of society.

 Take Action!

❖ Perform a functional analysis of your body. How can you accommodate the needs of your body so you can do the things you want and need to do?

❖ Stay in contact with your doctor, visiting at least once a year. Not only are new treatments being discovered, but it's also necessary to keep your doctor aware of your current condition, especially if you are receiving disability benefits.

❖ If you cannot work, seek out other ways to connect with and contribute to your community.

Budget Basics

Chronic pain often results in money problems. Doctors, tests, medications, and transportation to those things all take money. Many times, chronic pain leads to the loss of work, which puts an even greater strain on the wallet. Financial challenges can wreak havoc with your relationships and your emotions, while diminishing your recreational and medical options.

My Teacher's answer to economic difficulties was simple: Make more money. This worked well for me at first, when my body was healthy and strong. I was able to pay off my student loans and credit card debt, and even put money into a savings account. Through my career as a computer consultant, I experienced living without concern for money for the first time in my life. Finally not surviving paycheck to paycheck, my worry over lack of money dissipated. It was wonderful. As a Buddhist monk, my material needs were few, but it still comforted me to know I could afford anything I needed and still have money left to help others.

When my illness progressed to the point where I could no longer work, everything changed. This philosophy of making more money to cover my increasing medical expenses no longer applied because my body would not cooperate. I certainly tried to earn as much money as possible, however the body revolted and finally collapsed. I lost my job and lived on my savings, determined to go back to work within a month or two. Two months turned into three, and my doctors pushed the idea of applying for disability. Unfortunately, accepting disability income became the only reasonable choice.

Living on a fixed income, on disability, is a different life-style than working in the world. The option to get a raise or a higher paying job disappears. Two options remain: go deeper and deeper into debt, or learn how to budget your money to live within your means.

Much like pacing, living on a budget is a form of mindfulness: you consciously choose how to spend every penny that comes into your possession. Instead of buying products on a whim, you carefully choose what is going to benefit your life the most.

You take the time to shop for the best price. Money is really a form of power, of energy. How you spend your money is your choice, just as how you spend your energy is also your choice. You can spend your energy worrying about money, and pushing an idea of lack into your world, or you can direct that same power by making a conscious choice about your spending. When thoughts of worry arise, you will be able to push them out because you are honestly spending your money in the best possible way.

Following are the steps I took to create and manage a budget for myself. Please feel free to modify them to fit your particular situation.

1. Make a list of all of your expenses. Be sure to include everything – even the cup of coffee you buy at the shop down the street on your morning

walk. Also include the bills that come due every six months or once a year, like car registration and insurance.

2. Make a list of all your debt. Include the total amount, the interest rate, and the minimum payment due each month.

3. Write down your monthly income.

When you first write down all of your expenses, it can feel quite overwhelming, which is why many people avoid it like the plague. As you write down your expenses, remember to breathe. You don't need to solve all of your financial issues in this moment; all you're doing is setting up a plan so you can tackle those issues in a systematic way. When I made my first list, I cried when I was done. I couldn't believe how much money went through my hands each month. I double-checked my list and my math, and found that I missed a few things. I cried some more. Then I meditated. And with a clear mind, I went back to the list to see where I could realistically cut my spending.

A spreadsheet program like Excel is a useful tool to easily organize this information, and it will do the math for you. You may also want to track your spending in a money-management program like Quicken, which has a screen set up like a checkbook register and allows you to assign a category to the money you've spent. At the end of the month, you can run a report with all of your expenses itemized, added, and sorted into categories. You may be surprised at how much you actually spend on groceries, gifts to charity, and miscellaneous items.

If you do not have access to these programs, you can save all of your receipts (and be sure to either get a receipt or make a note for every penny you spend) for an entire month. Then organize the receipts into categories and add them up. Tracking every penny you pay out for several months is the best way to get an accurate picture of your spending. Be sure to include the things you consider a one-time purchase; you'd be surprised how quickly "miscellaneous" spending adds up.

For bills that are not due monthly, divide the amount due by the number of months in between payments. So if a bill is due every 6 months, divide it by 6. If it is due yearly, divide it by 12. The plan is to have the money available when the bill becomes due. This will allow you to avoid late fees and the transaction fees if you pay in installments. Look carefully at companies that offer an installment plan; some transaction fees can be as much as $10 per month if you select the installment option!

Your monthly list of expenses may look something like the one below. Please note I've simplified it to include only a few categories to make the math simple. Your actual list will have many more than are shown here.

CATEGORY	MONTHLY AMOUNT
Rent	500
Grocery	300
Auto:Insurance	50
Credit Cards	50
Clothes	0
TOTAL	900

After you create your list of actual expenses, you'll need to compare the Total to the amount of income you receive each month. If your income is less than your expenses, you'll need to do some cutting to bring everything into balance.

Reducing expenses is never an easy task. It can be fraught with emotion, so be sure to give yourself plenty of time to process what you need to do. This is the point where many people give up on the entire budgeting process, and they let themselves shut down mentally. Instead of giving into despair, take some time to meditate and then look at the numbers again.

Balancing your budget may require you to make sacrifices, like moving to a less expensive home, or buying cheaper groceries. Start by making a list of your absolute must-have expenses, like medication, food, rent, and transportation. Take an honest look at your grocery spending: Are you buying items on sale? Are you buying $10 steaks instead of $3 chicken for dinner? Also look closely at your "miscellaneous" spending; buying even a few cups of coffee each week at a restaurant can add up over time.

If you cannot meet your basic needs, there may be assistance available. Many drug companies offer free or low cost prescriptions to low-income people; check the manufacturer's website or ask your pharmacist for the manufacturer's phone number. You also may be eligible for government support for food and housing; check with your local government office.

When you first start managing your budget, if you have not been putting aside money for a bill that is coming due, you will need to catch-up for a while. For example, if you pay for car insurance every six months, and the next payment is due in two months, you will need to put extra money into your car insurance section when you build your budget management worksheet.

Let's say your car insurance is $300, so you will first divide that by 6, which equals $50 per month. Because the bill is due in two months, you will need to put an additional $100 per month aside for the next two months, for a total of $150 per month. Once you pay the $300 in car insurance, then your budget will change, and you'll put aside only $50 per month for insurance.

Subtract your total monthly expenses from your income to determine how much you can put in variable categories like: Clothes and Grocery. If you have money left over, you may want to add another category: Savings or Retirement. In an ideal situation, you'll put enough money to cover at least three months' worth of expenses aside in a savings account for unexpected events. If you are new to budgeting, this is a long-term goal you can work towards.

Use your list to create a monthly budget management worksheet, with the amount to put towards the categories every month. Each month will then have 3 columns to track your budget:

- Saved – the money you put into that category at the beginning of the month. On the first of the month, split up your income into categories, being sure you are not putting more into all the categories than you actually have on hand. Use the expense list you created previously to determine the amounts.

- Paid Out – the money you spent during the month for that category.

- Total – the amount you have left for future bills in that category at the end of the month.

In the example below, note that the Total for each month will be included in the Total from the previous month: First add the previous month's Total to Saved, and then subtract what you Paid Out to get your new month's Total. In our example, we are starting with zero in each category, and then going forward into January, we add 0 + SAVED – PAID OUT = TOTAL. We'll do this for each row. In February, we add January's TOTAL + SAVED – PAID OUT = February's TOTAL. We need to add only the TOTAL column at the end of each month.

I typically fill in the worksheet at the end of each month; however if your money is very tight, you can enter the SAVED amount at the beginning of the month or when you deposit money into your bank account, and then enter the PAID OUT during the month each time you pay out money in that category, and update the TOTAL each time. This will allow you to keep a close eye on how much is left in each category and adjust your spending as needed throughout the month.

CATEGORY	January			February			March		
	Saved	Paid Out	Total	Saved	Paid Out	Total	Saved	Paid Out	Total
Rent	500	500	0	500	500	0	500	500	0
Grocery	300	250	50	300	325	25	300	300	25
Auto:Insurance	150	0	150	150	0	300	50	300	50
Credit Cards	50	50	0	50	50	0	100	100	0
Clothes	0	0	0	0	0	0	50	25	25
TOTAL			200			325			100

Notice that the example above does not have all the categories you will, like medical expenses and gas & service for the car. I did this to keep the math simple. Keeping track of the money you allotted for a category but didn't spend will help you cover variable expenses like Grocery. In the chart above, the Paid Out amount for Grocery was more than we budgeted in February. Since we had money left over from January, we were able to pay the bills without any hardship.

In March, we paid the car insurance and reduced our Saved amount to 50 because now we have 6 months before the next payment is due. Because we no longer have to put extra money towards the car insurance, we added money to the Clothes and Credit Cards categories.

Use the Total/Total box at the very bottom to remind you how much money in your checking account is already budgeted for an expense. This will prevent you from thinking you have more money available than you actually do. In our example above, at the end of February we had a total of $325. We know from our budget worksheet that $300 is for the car insurance bill, which will arrive in March, and we have an extra $25 allocated for groceries.

In your budget, add categories like Travel & Gifts or Cash to save up for holidays and to give yourself a treat once in a while.

Once you create and maintain a monthly budget, your money stress will lessen. As you learn to live using a budget, you'll never find yourself wondering if you have enough money to buy a new shirt, or feeling guilty about giving yourself an extra treat. Instead, you will have the information you need about your finances to make a mindful decision about how you spend your money.

Two Common Issues With Debt:

My credit card debt is overwhelming and blowing my budget. What can I do?

If you have good credit, do everything you can to keep it. This will provide you with more options in the long run. Look at your list of debt, the interest rates, and the minimum payment. Over time, a lower interest rate means you'll pay less for the money you've borrowed. However, if you cannot pay more than the minimum payment, you are on the edge of trouble. If you miss a payment, the interest rate on your account may go up dramatically. In some cases, if you pay only minimum due each month on credit cards it will take 15 to 20 years to pay off the debt!

The first thing to do is stop using your credit cards that have a balance due. Ideally, you'll have one card that does not have a balance due. Use this card for convenience, but make sure you pay it off completely every month.

Then take your list of credit card debt (with the interest rate, balance, and minimum payment) and figure out how much you can pay in total towards your credit card debt. Pay more towards the balances that have the highest interest rate first. If the interest rate is the same on multiple cards, pay more towards the card with the balance that is closest to your credit limit. Having credit available will help improve your credit score, whereas having cards maxed-out will reduce your score.

Talk to your credit card companies and ask if they can give you a reduced interest rate. If you have a good credit score, companies may offer very low rates to get or keep your business. Ideally, you want a rate that will be fixed until the balance is paid off. If you transfer your balance to another credit card, be sure to ask about any fees and what the minimum payment will be, as the minimum payment can vary among companies. Also, if there is a fee to transfer your balance, ask what interest rate will be applied to the fee and when your payment will be applied to that fee as opposed to the transferred balance.

When considering a balance transfer, take the cost of fee into account when determining if it will save you money. Most credit card statements now show how much interest you'll pay on a balance over several years, which can help you see what your debt really costs. Sometimes changing to a zero percent promotion actually costs more because of the upfront transfer fee.

If you move your balance to a promotional rate that expires, mark your calendar two or three months ahead of the expiration date so you can find another offer. Once you accept any type of promotional rate, it's best not to use the card. If you use that credit card, the purchase will be charged at the standard rate, but your payment may be applied to the lower, promotional rate. This will cause you to rack up a lot of finance charges very quickly. Recent legislation has changed the rules credit card companies must follow when applying payments, so read your contract and any updates carefully if you do need to use a card with a promotional balance on it.

Once again, pay attention to the transfer fee, since that fee can reduce any savings you get from a lower interest rate.

As you shop for the best credit card, keep in mind that opening a new account may lower your credit score because part of the formula used is the average age of all your accounts. If you have had a credit card for ten years and then open a new one, the average age of your accounts will be reduced from ten to five. Most companies want to keep their customers, so talk to them about what offer you've found from others, and they may being willing to match it.

Another option is to talk to your local banks and credit unions to determine if a personal loan will work better for you. In some cases you may wind up paying a higher interest rate, but if the monthly payment fits your budget, you'll have a lower chance of ruining your credit. With personal loans, the payment period is set, so you'll know in four or five years, the loan will be paid off.

My credit rating is bad because I've fallen behind on my debt. What can I do?

Start by creating a personal budget and following the steps as noted above. Next, obtain a copy of your credit report from the three reporting agencies. You can get a free copy from www.AnnualCreditReport.com once per year. Check the reports for errors and follow their instructions to correct them.

This website also has information about repairing your credit in their Frequently Asked Questions section, and is an excellent resource. While there are many companies advertising services to help you fix your credit, you can typically do everything they can do for yourself at no cost. Ask your bank or credit union for tips on improving your credit score.

If you're having trouble making payments, work first on the debt that is current, meaning your payments haven't been late or sent to a collection agency. It looks better on your credit report to have never been late on some accounts than to be late on all of them. In other words, if you've always paid one account on time, do everything you can to stay current with that one.

Take the time to figure out what you can realistically pay towards each debt, including the ones you have fallen behind on. Then present your proposed payment plan to each company, and be prepared to compromise. Explain your situation clearly, and talk to a manager if necessary. Always try to do this before you miss a payment. You may need to agree to not use the card any longer. Again, ask for a reduced interest rate to help you get out of debt faster. Be extremely polite, even if they are not.

Companies would rather work with you to pay off your debt than send your account into collections. If the person you speak to on the phone cannot help you, try not to get upset. Instead ask to speak with a manager, or hang up and call back so you can talk to a different person; some credit card employees are easier to deal with than others.

If you begin to get frustrated, tell them you'll call them back. Take the time to practice meditation and mindfulness to pull yourself back into a higher mind state. Then get back on the phone with a brighter, more positive attitude.

If your debt has already gone to a collection agency, realize they probably paid much less for your loan than what you owe on it. Many times they paid pennies on the dollar for the right to collect your loan. Because of this, they may be willing to settle your debt completely for much less than you owe. Don't be afraid to negotiate with them.

Keep in mind that most negative information (a debt you did not pay or made late payment towards) remains on your credit report for 7 to 10 years. The time limit begins at the date of the last payment you made on the account. Although bankruptcy is typically removed from your credit report after 10 years, most loan applications and rental agreements I've filled out ask: "Have you ever filed bankruptcy?" so it's best to avoid bankruptcy in most cases. Ideally, you'll pay off all of your debt eventually. However, because of the time limit on negative reporting, it's a good idea to make current payments on your most recent debt since it will affect your credit score longer than old debt.

One exception to the 10-year rule is any debt that was backed by the government, such as a student loan. This type of debt will remain, and the government has the right to collect it from you, and can take it out of your social security checks and/or federal tax refunds. The best thing to do is contact them and work out a payment plan. Be sure you have your budget information in front of you when you speak to them. They will be more likely to listen if you give exact details of your expenses and income rather than telling them you just can't pay.

Decide how many credit cards you really need,

and if you have too many, close the newest ones first. Unless the credit cards are a temptation for you, keep one or two of your older accounts open, and once they are paid off use them occasionally to keep them active. Be sure to pay the balance in full each time you use it to avoid getting in trouble again. And of course, always read any changes in terms whenever they are announced.

If you decide to work with a credit counselor, be sure you fully understand all of the costs involved before you sign anything. Check with the Better Business Bureau (www.bbb.org) and the Federal Trade Commission (www.ftc.gov) to make sure the company you're dealing with is reputable.

While it does take energy, it's worth the time to try to resolve your credit problems on your own before you approach one of these companies. As you work on tackling your debt, practice mindfulness. Whenever you feel frazzled, step back to center yourself and clear your mind.

Taking responsibility for your debt and making an effort to resolve it is a very empowering act. Instead of being pushed around by others, it's an opportunity for you to make the financial decisions that will help create the best possible future for you.

Take Action!

❖ If you're not quite ready to tackle your budget today, keep a money diary for a month. Use a spreadsheet program like Excel (or download LibreOffice for free) to record your spending every day. If you cannot get on the computer every day, then use a notebook and type it in later or add it up with a calculator. Write down where you spent the money (grocery store or restaurant, etc.) and how much. Be sure to count every dollar that leaves your hand.

❖ Much more information about budgeting is available; you can do a search on the internet for "personal budget" for free worksheets and other methods. For example, Mint.com offers a free app to track your budget on your smart phone or computer.

❖ Schedule time to begin work on your budget. Also add in a time each month to maintain your budget worksheet once you've created one.

❖ If you share finances with someone else, talk openly about the budget. If things begin to get heated, take a break. Being able to discuss money issues without emotions getting in the way is an important part of any long-term relationship.

❖ Look for entertainment options that are low cost or free. For example, many large cities have free museum days for local residents.

❖ Be mindful of how stress about money affects you mentally and physically. Instead of ignoring it, take action by consciously managing your spending.

Treatments And Therapies
(A Limited List)

New treatments are discovered every day. Not all of them work for everyone. Treating chronic pain is very much a trial and error process for every individual. When living with chronic pain for a long time, most people go through a sense of desperation where they are willing to try anything for any price to gain some relief. Unfortunately, there are thousands of people out there waiting to take advantage of someone in a state of desperation. They will promise you complete relief, for only $5000. Some people buy into it, and that's why these con artists continue to look for new targets. The placebo effect, where something works purely because you believe it will, can be very powerful. Unfortunately, it often wears off, leaving you in the same amount of pain and your wallet a little lighter.

Some of the products available through the Internet actually do help some. However, if someone promises you complete relief at a huge cost, be cautious. There's nothing wrong with investigating the latest and greatest nutritional or herbal products, or the healing devices available on the market. However, always do your research and use your common sense. Miracles happen every day, but they usually don't cost $59.95 plus shipping and handling.

The first place to seek treatment is with your

doctor. Be sure to ask questions if he or she gives you a recommendation. Understand what the treatment involves, how it will help, and any possible side effects. When you decide to go ahead with the treatment (remember it is your choice!), pay close attention to how it affects you. If you experience something unexpected, call your doctor right away to find out what you should do. And once again, use your common sense.

Be aware that some doctors (and/or secretaries) have trouble listening to patients who have unusual side effects. Your pharmacist and drug information websites like www.RXList.com are excellent resources for you to investigate the medications your doctor may prescribe.

As you begin your experiments to discover the best treatment plan for you, take it slow and take notes for yourself. Keep a folder or notebook of past treatments; don't expect your health care providers to keep this information for you.

Try each new treatment one at a time, giving each one at least a week to see how it affects your pain, your body and your mind. If you try three different treatments at the same time, and you start to feel better, you'll have no way of knowing which one is working. Alternatively, if you feel worse, you also won't know which one to stop. Trying treatments one by one is time consuming and can be frustrating. However, a systematic approach will give you the most information in the shortest amount of time.

Keep a list of the things you've tried and the effect they had, so you don't forget and start repeating the same thing over again.

Some health care providers can be very pushy when it comes to recommending treatments. Always be aware that you have the final say on your treatment plan. Listen carefully to your doctors, and decide what is best for you. If a recommended treatment doesn't sound right, express your concerns immediately. There may be something either you or your doctor does not understand about your situation.

To avoid being labeled an uncooperative patient when refusing a treatment, be clear to your doctor about why you do not want to explore that treatment right now. It's always OK to say you want to try something else first, and if you run out of options, then you'll consider the one he recommended. If the doctor tells you there's only one treatment and you do not agree with it, consult with a different doctor. It's not worth your energy to argue with a doctor who cannot or will not work with you to find treatments that help.

When you find a treatment that helps some, but you're still in pain, then add new treatments to the one you've found. Again, use the one by one approach. You may, over time, find a combination of treatments that help enough for you to have a more active lifestyle.

You may need to give yourself a break from the experiments once in a while. Stop and go have fun in whatever way you can. Not knowing how your body will be feeling from day to day is a tough way to live. Stopping for a while so you can better predict what you can do is important because then you can make plans to go out with friends. When you're ready, pick up where you left off. Above all else, never give up.

Take Action!

❖ Create a folder or notebook for doctor appointments. It should contain your current medications and treatments. Make a section for past treatments and note how they affected you. Keep in mind treatments include medication, dietary and lifestyle changes, exercise, body work, and more.

❖ Make a separate section for treatment options you may want to learn more about or explore in the future.

❖ After every doctor appointment, or after trying a new treatment, take five or ten minutes to update your folder.

Nutrition

"If you don't eat, you die."
~Jim Sundell

Food has an amazing effect on the human body. All the things you put in your mouth are literally the building blocks for every cell in your body. Even chewing an ordinary stick of gum releases sugar into your blood stream. Our diet is probably the one thing we have the most control over, yet it can be the most difficult thing to change. The body and digestive system have become accustomed to the food you eat; change too much too fast and it will have a negative reaction.

When you live in chronic pain, your body is burning up a great deal of energy because of the pain. You're probably too exhausted to cook a gourmet meal, so you grab whatever is easy and convenient. You may even skip meals because you are too tired. It's important to remember the less nutrition you give your body, the less energy it will have.

The easiest thing to give your body is high quality water. This should be common sense, but if you feel thirsty, that means your body needs water. By staying well hydrated your entire body functions better. If you drink more than 3 cups of coffee or soda in a day, the caffeine can dehydrate you. Many medications can contribution to dehydration as well. Make it a practice to always have a glass or bottle of water with you all day long. After a week or two, you'll probably start to notice the difference.

If you are not lucky enough to live in an area with high quality tap water, purchase a filtration system or bottled water. Some people are very sensitive to the additives in tap water; others are even sensitive to filtered water. If the bottle is not marked "Spring Water" then it is mostly likely filtered tap water.

Keep bottles out of the sun; the sun reacts with the plastic and can give the water a nasty taste and you a belly ache, and may have other serious health consequences. Pure water is essential to everyone's health, and for a person with chronic pain it can mean the difference between a tolerable day and a horrible one.

Some people don't like water because they are not accustomed to drinking it, or it may be the temperature. You may find it easier to drink water at room temperature, or you may prefer it cold or warm. If you still cannot get yourself to drink plain water, add a teaspoon of fruit juice or honey to a full glass for flavor. The grocery store has many varieties of designer "water" – read the labels carefully before purchasing them. Many are full of sugar and additives.

While you're at the grocery store, remember to pick up simple foods, which require little to no preparation so you can eat something good for you when you're exhausted. Soup is an excellent choice; you don't even have to chew to eat it! There are many high quality microwave dinners on the market for those really bad days. Be sure to keep lots of healthy snacks around; cheese, sliced vegetables, fruit, and crackers are some great examples.

Many people find they feel better if they eat four to five small meals each day. With smaller portions, the digestive system doesn't need to work as hard, and your body has a steady supply of energy all day long. This practice also makes you stop every couple of hours, even if it is just to eat. A diet high in protein is beneficial to many people with chronic pain; however do not neglect the other foods groups as they provide important building blocks for your body.

Your doctor may want to test you for nutritional deficiencies. Low magnesium and DHEA levels are often found in Fibromyalgia patients. Other tests may include calcium, vitamin D, and iron levels. If you do test low, be sure to have your doctor re-test you after you begin using supplements, to make certain your body is absorbing them. Over the counter supplements are not regulated the same way as prescription drugs are, so stick with reliable suppliers.

Hypoglycemia (low-blood sugar) and diabetes can both cause intense fatigue, so it's worth asking your doctor about those diseases to see if they are contributing to your health issues.

Another condition to discuss with your doctor is food allergy or sensitivity. Some researchers claim that most of the population is sensitive to at least one or more widely consumed food products. A genuine allergy is typically easy to spot: swelling, hives, or itching within minutes of eating the problem food. However, food sensitivity often goes undetected. Some common problem foods include soy (hormone and emotional disturbances), gluten (everything from snoring to fatigue to stomach aches), and milk products (diarrhea and cramps).

If you begin eating a new food and notice a new symptom, the easiest thing to do is avoid the new food and see if your symptom goes away. Once the symptom is completely gone, try eating the suspected food again to see if the symptom comes back. You'll need to ensure you are getting the nutrients from another source while you avoid that food.

For people who think they may have food sensitivities but do not know which foods are to blame, the best course of action is to discuss your situation with a nutritionist. Unfortunately the only way to know for certain if food sensitivity is a problem is to go on an elimination diet. Elimination diets can be very risky because without proper dietary knowledge, you may not get all the nutrition you need. Without proper nutrition, you'll end up feeling worse than when you started, so there will be no way to tell if the suspect food is actually a problem. Do some research and talk to your doctor before attempting this process.

Organic and all-natural foods have been shown to be helpful for people with a variety of medical conditions. While they still tend to be a bit more expensive, they are becoming easier to find in local stores as people become more conscious about the negative impact of pesticides and chemicals in our food.

There are many wonderful books about the benefits of organic and all-natural foods you can read to learn more. You can begin to make a shift to healthier eating today by reading the ingredients of the foods you plan to buy. Once you become aware of what's actually in your favorite bag of chips, you may decide to try something new.

Be mindful of what you put in your mouth every day. If you are not eating a healthy diet now, begin today to improve. Paying attention is the first step. Then start small, like adding more vegetables to each meal or eating fruit as a snack instead of a cookie.

Give your mind and body time to adjust to the change. You'll be more successful if you change your eating habits gradually, rather than suddenly denying yourself all of your favorite foods and replacing them with things unfamiliar to your digestive track.

Remember, it won't help anyone if you beat yourself up for eating the wrong foods; instead congratulate yourself each time you make a healthy food choice. One day you may find eating healthy has become a natural, normal way of life for you.

 Take Action!

- ❖ Increase your fruit and vegetables to at least 5 servings a day. If you haven't been eating any fruits and vegetables, start by adding one per day.

- ❖ Juice Plus® is a whole-food supplement that can help increase your fruit and vegetable intake. More information about this product can be found on the Internet.

- ❖ Experiment with different foods; try a new, healthy food product once a week.

Body Work

Chronic pain can bind up your muscles and tendons, making you feel like you cannot do anything. Simply eating a meal may cause intolerable pain. Sitting through a two hour movie may hurt long after you leave the theater. When the pain is this bad (or even if it isn't) a good body worker can do wonders for your functionality.

Like everything else, body workers vary in expertise, style, and personality. Before giving up on a type of bodywork, try a different therapist. Always ask questions when you make the appointment so you know what to expect. There are thousands of schools, and they train their students differently. The body workers who graduate from those schools also have their own interests; some want to only help people relax while others want to help treat medical conditions. Within the group who want to help people with chronic pain, some body workers have more experience dealing with certain problems than others. Take the time to research and find someone who is a good match for your particular condition and your personality.

My first physical therapist treated my chronic illness like a simple muscle injury. She had me exercise in a pool and then gave me some exercises to do at home. She asked me to call her when I had recovered from the first treatment. A week later, she called me wondering why I had not called. She had me return for another treatment a few days later. After each visit, my condition grew worse and worse. Even though I complained right away about the negative impact of the treatment, she changed only the length of time and not the exercises. After the fourth and final visit, she told me to have my doctor adjust my medications. She insisted the treatment she prescribed was what worked for my condition, even though it had obviously done more harm than good.

It took a couple of years before I was ready to try physical therapy again. When I decided I had enough control over my pain to try again, I called several physical therapists and asked about their treatment plan. Most offered what I had already tried. I kept calling and finally found one who offered a different approach, which eventually did improve my endurance. I also went through several massage therapists, acupuncturists and chiropractors before I found the ones that provide positive results for my body. I continue to explore the different types of bodywork available in my quest for improved functionality.

As you begin your own search, remember to ask questions before committing to treatment. Most therapists are happy to talk you on the phone if you have specific questions. After you begin, continue to evaluate if the treatment is increasing your functionality and helping you feel better. Please keep in mind most bodywork treatments do not cure illness; rather they improve the quality of your life by helping you minimize pain and other symptoms. Personally, I would be very skeptical of anyone claiming to cure me, especially if their treatments are very expensive and they do not accept insurance.

Some questions to consider:

- How long have you been in practice?
- Have you treated others with chronic pain from: [your condition]?
- What were their outcomes?
- What is your treatment plan for someone with my condition?
- How many treatments do you expect me to need to have results?
- Do you accept insurance? How much do you charge per treatment?

Remember, you know your body best. Although we would like to think one treatment works for everyone, it simply doesn't. It's easy to give up your care to a trusted professional; however chronic problems usually require more attention than the one-size-fits-all outlook of many therapists. Keep exploring to find the body workers who can help you get the most functionality out of your body as possible.

Physical Therapy

Types of physical therapy vary widely among therapists. Some offer only exercises designed to strengthen muscles. Others incorporate either active or passive stretching into their routines. A few use Hatha Yoga or Tai Chi movements as part of a treatment plan. Still fewer use manual therapy, where they move your joints through the range of motion and may also incorporate various types of massage. The use of tools such as ultrasound, electrical stimulation, and hot or cold packs is also common.

Active stretching is where you use your muscles to stretch the surrounding muscles. Passive stretching uses gravity to achieve a stretch. To do a passive stretch, you may use pillows or special tables that allow the muscle to hang down, thus causing a gentle stretch.

Any type of stretch, active or passive, should never hurt. There should only be a gentle pulling sensation. If a stretch hurts, it will cause the muscles to tighten in reaction to the pain. This reaction is an automatic response, which allows the muscle to protect itself. If you continue to stretch to the point of pain, the muscle may create a knot or trigger point, keeping the muscles tight even when at rest.

In the beginning, you may be able to do a proper stretch with only a few millimeters of movement. If you practice every day, you will slowly improve and be able to stretch further and expand your range of motion. Be mindful every time you stretch so you do not put yourself in more pain.

A good physical therapist can give you ways to incorporate exercises and stretches appropriate for your condition into your daily life. Communicate clearly with your physical therapist each time you see him or her. If an exercise or stretch you have been given hurts, make sure the therapist understands that you know the difference between it being slightly uncomfortable and outright painful. Pain means you're pushing too far. You may need to go home and rest after a visit, but it should not wipe you out for weeks. The goal is not to torture yourself; the goal is to improve your functionality.

Biofeedback & Relaxation Techniques

Biofeedback is used by some therapists to help you gain an awareness of your muscle tension. When we feel pain, the muscles in the body automatically contract. Constantly contracted muscles create even more pain. The cycle continues until the body becomes too tight to move at all and you feel like one big ball of pain.

A biofeedback machine assigns a number to the tension level of the muscle to which it is attached. You can see the number on the screen and compare it to how you feel. As you sit hooked up to the machine, you practice consciously relaxing the muscle. When you are successful, the number drops. This device is an objective way for you to measure muscle tension and helps you become aware of how you feel when your muscles are not as contracted.

At home, you continue the practice by rating your muscle tension on a chart throughout the day. The therapist will have you rate your muscle tension right before hooking you up to the machine so you can see how accurate you are.

By being aware of your muscle tension on a constant basis, you can learn to control it and reduce your tension-based pain levels. This is a practice of mindfulness applied to the muscles of the body. Although it not a cure-all, it is a powerful tool you can use to dramatically reduce the negative effects of chronic muscle tension on your body.

When a therapist teaches you Biofeedback, they often include relaxation techniques. Relaxation exercises are different from meditation. In meditation, you are expanding your awareness. During meditation the body does relax, however that is not its primary purpose. With relaxation techniques, you are simply relaxing your body and letting your mind wander. Here are three easy relaxation techniques you can try on your own:

1. Lie down on a comfortable couch or bed. Then beginning with the top of your head and stretching down to your face, concentrate on each muscle by visualizing a soft white light around it. Keep focusing and breathing into each muscle until it slightly softens. Move your focus down the back of your head to your neck, repeating the visualization while taking slow breaths. Then move into your shoulders and down your arms slowly. Continue to move all the way down your torso, taking the time to relax your chest, back, and pelvis before moving down the legs. Relax your toes, allowing all the tension to exit at the bottom of your feet. If you feel like you need to stretch or wiggle a muscle, allow yourself to do so. Give yourself plenty of time; this cannot be rushed. Whenever you have trouble sleeping, this is a wonderful technique to use while lying in bed.

2. To relieve pressure in your legs and back, lie down or sit with your legs supported and move your ankles in small circles. Then change the direction and move your ankles in the opposite direction.

3. For tight shoulders, stand up and bend slightly towards the left, allowing your left arm to hang

down your side. Support yourself with your other arm against a wall if you feel unsteady. Let your arm hang down until it begins to move – all by itself – in circles. Let your arm unwind itself; eventually the direction of the circles will change, again it will do it by itself. Don't try to force the circles. You may need to let your arm hang for a few minutes before it moves. Then repeat the process on the right arm. This technique works especially well in a hot shower.

One popular technique to be cautious with is "progressive relaxation" because it may cause more pain in some people. When I tried it during a pain management class and again when I listened to a relaxation CD someone gave me, it completely backfired. This technique involves tightening and then releasing the muscles one by one. This is supposed to cause a deeper level of relaxation. However with me, the muscles became stuck in a state of contraction when I tightened them. So when I tried this technique, I was not able to relax the muscles. Instead my entire body became stuck in a state of contraction that lasted for several hours. If you are inclined to try it, experiment first with a small area of your body and wait a few hours before trying more to see how your body reacts.

Relaxation techniques are an important tool for anyone with chronic pain, even if you do not have the opportunity to work with a Biofeedback therapist. While the first response for many people is to get annoyed when someone tells them to relax, consciously relaxing your muscles to the best of your ability does relieve some of the pain. The majority of the pain may still be present, however lowering the levels by even one notch is worth the effort. As an added benefit, the more relaxed you are, the clearer your mind will be, thus allowing you to make better decisions regarding your health and your life.

Acupuncture

Acupuncture is an ancient form of Oriental Medicine, and often involves the use of both tiny needles and herbs. There are many different styles of acupuncture. From my experience, Chinese acupuncture is more aggressive than Japanese style acupuncture. The Chinese style uses slightly larger needles and more insertion sites, while the Japanese style seems to have a more subtle approach.

Acupuncturists are more concerned with finding root causes than treating symptoms. The acupuncturist may have you fill out a questionnaire and ask you about things that do not seem related to your problem. They may even want to look at your tongue to help them determine their treatment plan. (The tongue is the only muscle visible without cutting into the body.) The terms used by an acupuncturist are often unfamiliar to the Western ear. When an acupuncturist takes your pulse, they may describe it with odd words such as wiry, deficient, or slippery. During treatment, the needles may cause strange sensations in your body as your "chi" is moved into balance.

Although I do not have a deep understanding of this approach to medicine, I have found it to be tremendously effective. After only a few treatments with the right therapist, I experienced a reduction of pain and an improved sense of well-being. For me, the effects so far have not been permanent; however others I know have found a lasting benefit. Whenever I see my acupuncturist for a treatment session, I always leave feeling better than when I walked in.

Massage

I once thought massage was only for spoiled rich people who spent all day lounging at a Day Spa drinking wine. Before that, I had an even lower opinion: a masseuse was just another name for a prostitute. Fortunately both of these uninformed attitudes were completely wrong. Massage therapy is actually one of the most beneficial types of bodywork available.

There are many types of massage therapy, so researching your options is an important first step. Insurance typically does not pay for massage therapy; however don't let cost be the only deciding factor when selecting a therapist. Some physical therapists offer massage as a part of their treatment program, so your insurance may pay for it in this situation.

When making an appointment, ask the therapist if he or she has experience treating patients who have your health condition. Deep tissue massage works well for releasing trigger points, however it typically makes Fibromyalgia pain worse. In my experience, a massage that concentrates on improving circulation in the deeper muscles works well for Fibromyalgia.

When you are receiving a massage, communicate with the therapist about the pressure. If it's too strong, or if the technique she's using is causing irritation, speak up right away. Massage therapists are trained in a variety of techniques, but they won't know to try something different until you tell them.

CranioSacral massage is a specific type of treatment I have found to be very helpful during severe pain flares, when even a light touch hurts. It's probably the gentlest technique I have experienced; yet it is profoundly powerful. During a CranioSacral session, you lay down fully clothed on a massage table. The therapist uses pressure points at the base of the spine, the skull, and other various points to relieve pain and shift the body back into its natural alignment. It is especially useful for people with disc problems. Many people fall asleep during the treatment, and wake up refreshed. With this technique, always look for a therapist with advanced training.

If money is tight, an option is to call the local massage schools. They often have programs where students give massages at very low prices. Keep in mind that you will need to be extremely vocal about what is working and what is not during the massage. Students do not have the same skill level in reading body language as a more experienced therapist.

An independent massage therapist may be able to work with your budget, whereas a Day Spa has set prices. Day Spas charge you not only for the massage, but also for amenities like a locker room, hot tub, sauna, and steam room. Prices vary widely, so take the time to call around and ask questions.

Massage clubs are also becoming popular, where you sign a one-year contract to join. One massage per month is usually included in the monthly fee, and you'll receive additional massages at a reduced price. These clubs often offer a trial massage at a reduced rate.

After a massage, drink plenty of water. If possible, soak in a warm bath. Always plan your visit so you can rest for the remainder of the day, to give your body time to absorb the benefits of the massage.

Chiropractors

A chiropractor adjusts the joints within the body to bring it back into natural alignment. Some chiropractors adjust only the neck and spine, while others do adjustments throughout the body. There can be large differences among practitioners, so just as with other types of body workers, if the first one you see is not helpful, try another one.

Chiropractic care has become widely accepted in recent years, and many insurance plans, including Medicare, will pay for treatment of misalignment. Check with your plan to see if a referral from your primary care physician is required, and be sure to ask the chiropractor if they accept your insurance when you make the appointment. Some chiropractors offer a free evaluation to see if their treatment will help you; however, always ask about fees when you call.

Many chiropractors use hot packs and/or electric stimulation before or after a treatment to help relax the surrounding muscles. They may also recommend stretches for you to do at home. As with massage therapy, plan to rest after your visit.

While the actual adjustment can be painful, the

benefits often outweigh the temporary discomfort. A chiropractor can help to increase the range of motion in your neck and back, as well as decrease overall pain levels. Again, always ask questions, and if you are not getting the results you need from one chiropractor, try a different one.

Exercise

Pain can make it difficult to exercise; ironically, exercise can help reduce pain. The first minute or two, as the body pops and cracks, may make you want to stop right away. However, moving around reduces the pain caused by stiffness and can help unwind contracted muscles. Over time, regular exercise will also help to build your endurance for all activities.

The level at which you can exercise will vary depending upon the condition of your body on that particular day. You may be able to only walk around for three minutes before the pain becomes too intense. Three minutes is a fine place to start. Or, you may not be able to walk around; perhaps all you can do is wiggle your arms and turn at the waist for a minute or two. That's also a fine place to start. As with everything, you begin wherever you are.

Moving increases circulation, stretches muscles and tendons, and decreases mental fatigue. You don't need to run a marathon or lift weights at the local gym to exercise. There are many things you can do in your own home to get started.

Stretching is probably the best way to begin. A stretch should not be painful; rather it should feel like a very gentle tug.

From your chair, stretch your legs out. Now stretch your arms. Then try stretching your neck from one side to the other, and then by rotating your head in a circle. You may not be able to move very far today. Your neck may move only a few millimeters before it hurts. In this case, stretch your neck only a few millimeters; turn very slowly until you feel the gentle tug, hold it for a couple of breaths and then turn back to the center. One or two stretches in each direction is enough to start with; it's important not to do too many repetitions. If you stretch like this every day, your range of motion will improve, little by little.

There are several exercise classes I have found helpful: the Feldenkrais method, Hatha Yoga, and Tai Chi. A class can be wonderful not only for your body, but also for your mood since you'll have the opportunity to interact with others and learn something new.

A Feldenkrais Method instructor can teach you new ways of moving your body. By helping you to gain an awareness of what your body can do in its current state, you may find you can do much more than you realized. Simply changing how you perform an action may allow you to perform that action without increasing your pain. If you can afford to, private sessions are a wonderful addition to public classes since the teacher will be able to spend all of their time working directly with you.

Hatha Yoga, with the right instructor, can be very helpful. This form of yoga uses the body to help the mind achieve a state of peace. In the process, the muscles of the body become more flexible and stronger and the body finds its natural alignment. It looks easier than it actually is. An average class attracts many healthy people, and you may hurt yourself by trying to do too much too fast. Instead of going to the first class you find, look for an instructor with experience teaching people who have chronic pain. During class, be mindful of your own comfort zone to prevent yourself from pushing too hard.

Tai Chi is an ancient martial art and an excellent complement to meditation practice. Any type of martial art can give you a certain edge that helps you deal with all types of pain. Tai Chi is unique in that it is gentle enough for anyone to practice.

Through Tai Chi, you learn to use your entire body. Rather than depending upon your muscles for support, Tai Chi teaches you how to stand and move by using your bones for support. Over time, Tai Chi can help to improve your balance, flexibility, strength, concentration, and endurance.

There are many classes specially designed for people with chronic pain or for senior citizens that are a great place to start. Always notify your instructor about your condition, be mindful of your body, and respect your limits.

During any exercise session, sit or lay down to rest as often as you need to. Don't wait until your pain has become intense; at the first sign of a significant increase, stop and rest until you feel better. This may mean you participate for only a few minutes during each class, until you build up your endurance.

When I first began learning Tai Chi, I had to sit down every five minutes. Since I was the youngest person in class, I felt a little self-conscious about resting, but no one seemed to mind. Even years later, I still need to stop and rest often during class. When I do get up to continue, there is always a feeling of encouragement from the other students.

As you begin a new class, give yourself extra time to learn the routines. When I first learned the short form of Tai Chi, I had to concentrate on only one move each week. During my first week, I practiced the first move every day during television commercials. When my show came back on, I would rest until the next commercial. The following week, I learned the second movement. Then at home, I practiced the first two moves, during the television commercials. Some weeks I had to back up and relearn a move I didn't get. Other weeks I had to break down the new move and learn it over several weeks. I've been practicing for several years now, and although I continue to discover improvements in class each week, I've learned enough to go through the Short Form by myself. The flowing movements of Tai Chi are a wonderful way to get my body moving in the morning.

As you explore your options, you may find many videos that teach Tai Chi and Hatha Yoga that you can do at home in front of your television. Be careful as you practice, because without a teacher in the room with you, no one is checking your form. Neither of these exercises should cause an increase in pain. If something starts to hurt, your form may be incorrect. Keep the remote handy, so you can pause and rewind as necessary.

Another option for excising at home is the Nintendo Wii® video game. It offers fun, interactive sports like bowling, tennis, and golf. With the Wii Fit program, there are balance games, yoga poses, and aerobics. With any exercise you do on your own, remember to closely monitor your pain levels so you don't do too much.

In whatever way you can, treat yourself to some exercise every day. Take it slow, rest as much as you need to, and move your body each and every day.

Things You Can Do at Home

Not everyone who lives with chronic pain has access to the therapies and classes I've discussed. That doesn't mean you need to sit and suffer. In addition to the stretching and relaxation techniques described above, there are a few other things you can do to help alleviate some of the pain.

Invest in a good reusable hot pack or heating pad. Putting heat on an aching muscle can bring pain levels down from intense to tolerable. If you cannot afford a hot pack, you can make your own by heating a damp towel in the microwave. Be careful not to burn yourself. Also, do NOT put a towel in a conventional or toaster oven, since it may catch fire.

If your joints hurt and are warm, try an ice pack. Sometimes you may not be able to see the swelling of a joint, but you may feel it. You can also try alternating the hot and cold packs every ten minutes. Alternating heat and cold improves circulation and can help you feel better.

A warm bath is a wonderful way to soothe your entire body. Epsom salt, sea salts, mineral salts, and lavender oil are known for helping to relieve muscle soreness. If you don't have a bathtub, soak your feet in a large pan and relax.

Another option to investigate is Aromatherapy. Look for high-quality, all natural oils, keeping in mind a small amount goes a long way. Lavender oil applied to the skin is known for helping tight muscles relax.

 Take Action!

❖ Call your insurance company to learn what types of bodywork they cover, such as physical therapy, chiropractic care, acupuncture, biofeedback, or massage therapy.

❖ In your medical notebook, keep a list of the bodywork and exercises you've done and how they have impacted your pain and functionality.

❖ Begin each day with a few minutes of stretching.

❖ Do a little exercise each day, such as walking to the mailbox, up and down stairs, or around the block.

❖ If you cannot sleep, practice the relaxation techniques described in this chapter.

Medication

There are many medication options available for treating pain, and new ones are being discovered each year. All medication use, including over-the-counter products, should be discussed with your doctor. I have no medical training and can offer only my personal experiences. Your doctor knows the most about your particular condition and should be consulted before trying any type of medication, even if it does not require a prescription.

The most common drugs for treating chronic pain fall into these categories: anti-inflammatory, muscle-relaxant, anti-depressant, and opioid. Some doctors also prescribe anti-seizure medications like Neurontin, although it is not understood why they help with chronic pain. Lyrica, recently approved by the FDA for Fibromyalgia, was developed from this branch of pharmacology.

Medications may not stop all of the pain, however they may dull the pain enough for you to improve the quality of your life. When considering the use of any medication, you will need to evaluate for yourself if the relief it provides outweighs the side effects.

In addition to the physical effects of a medication, you also need to weigh the psychological ones. Discuss your medication use with a trusted friend or family member, as well as making notes in your own journal. Drugs sometimes can unexpectedly affect our personality and temperament. It can be difficult for the person taking the drug to notice these changes. If you notice anger, apathy, or other mental states unusual to you, talk to your friend and check your notes to be sure it's not a result of the medication.

Anti-inflammatory medications reduce swelling and typically have a pain-relieving effect. Many anti-inflammatory drugs are non-steroidal and can be purchased over the counter in low doses. (While steroid-type anti-inflammatory drugs are sometimes helpful in reducing pain, their side effects, including a lowered immune system, make them undesirable for long-term use.) For some people, this type of medication is enough to control their chronic pain. Non-steroidal anti-inflammatory drugs should always be taken with food to prevent serious stomach problems. These drugs may take up to two weeks for their full effect to be noticed.

Muscle-relaxant medications, like the name suggests, work on the central nervous system to relax the muscles and thus relieve muscle pain. Side effects can include dizziness, lack of motivation, and drowsiness. Some people notice a hangover effect when the medication has worn off, and this may last for a few days. Many people develop a tolerance to muscle-relaxants and must change to a different pill within the same class of drug.

Anti-depressant medications in very low doses have been found in FDA trials to help alleviate neuropathic (nerve) pain and Fibromyalgia symptoms for some of the people in the studies. They have also been found to provide relief for other chronic pain conditions and help people sleep through the night.

Unfortunately for me, these types of drugs were not helpful and created severe problems. Instead of making me sleepy, the anti-depressants caused agitation and I became wired for several days after discontinuing the medication. Apparently this has been reported from less than 1% of the population; however I have spoken with others who have had this same issue. I had this type of reaction to all the drugs I have tried within this class. However, these medications are worth investigating with your doctor since they have been proven to be helpful for some people with chronic pain. Because they affect brain-chemistry, use them with caution and be very aware of how you feel both physically and mentally while trying them.

Keep in mind if your doctor suggests anti-depressants, it doesn't necessarily mean he or she thinks you are depressed. When used to treat clinical depression, the doses are normally much higher than when these medications are used to treat chronic pain. Anti-depressant medication typically needs to build up in your system to reach therapeutic levels, so it may take a few weeks before you see any benefits. Of course, if you experience bothersome side-effects with any medication, contact your doctor immediately.

Opioid medications block the pain receptors in the brain, thus alleviating the sensation of pain. In a sense, opioid drugs stop the pain signals sent by the body from reaching the brain. If the body is not in a high degree of pain, there will be too much of the opioid in the system, which causes an experience of euphoria.

This euphoric sensation can be addictive psychologically. Any risk of addiction makes doctors nervous about prescribing opioid medication for long-term use. However, most chronic pain patients do not experience euphoria when taking this type of drug because their bodies are using it to block the pain. For this reason, the number of pain patients who become addicted to opioid medication is extremely low. According to a WebMD article by Eric Metcalf, only 3% of people taking opioids for non-cancer chronic pain became addicted, and the risk falls to less than 1% for people who never abused drugs.

If you feel "high" after taking an opioid, you're probably taking more than what you need and may want to reduce your dose. When using opioid drugs for pain relief, always take the lowest dose that provides relief. Keep in mind a pain reliever may not stop all of the pain; it may only make the pain more bearable.

When used long term, your body may become dependent upon opioid medication. Remember, there is a difference between being addicted and being dependent. With addiction, there is a psychological component that makes you think you must have the drug. When you are physically dependent upon a medication, you may experience withdrawal effects (like vomiting or profuse sweating) if you miss a couple of doses.

If opioid medication is required for an extended amount of time, some physicians recommend taking it on a schedule rather than on an as-needed basis. By taking doses at a set time each day, it removes the psychological connection of taking a pill to feel better and may help reduce the risk of addiction.

This type of meditation also works better if you take it before the pain becomes intense. Before making any changes to your medication usage, always discuss it with your doctor.

Another issue with opioid medication is tolerance. Tolerance means the same amount of medication no longer provides the same relief. The first thing to ask yourself is if you have been practicing your pacing and self care. Many times you may discover you are pushing yourself too hard, and this is causing an increase in your normal pain levels. Slowing down and taking time to care for yourself mentally and physically may be enough for the pain medication to provide relief again. However, if the things you try do not bring your pain down to manageable levels, then it's time to talk to your doctor about increasing the dosage of your medication.

An alternative to increasing your dose is to try a "drug holiday" where you wean yourself off the medication and then go without it for a few days or weeks. In preparation for a drug holiday, it's important to reduce your dose gradually – suddenly stopping an opioid medication can cause severe complications including seizures and permanent damage. **Before you start this process, you must discuss it with your doctor.** Part of your discussion is how long you will need to be completely off of the medication, as it will depend on how long and how much you have taken. Once the drug is out of your system, your body should not need as much medication to get relief when you start taking it again.

The drug holiday, while effective, can be very difficult. Talk with your doctor before attempting it and plan for the increased pain by making non-drug therapies easily available and resting the entire time.

(Please note: the "drug holiday" technique should not be done with anti-depressants, as they work better in the body by building up over time.) Your pharmacist can help you understand what to expect and confirm exactly how long it will take for the medication to completely leave your system, since this timeframe may vary among different drugs.

Some doctors are completely against the use of opioid medications. If you have tried everything else and nothing is helping enough for you to have a quality life, find another doctor. Nothing you say or do will convince these types of doctors to prescribe the medication to you. Attempting to do so may even backfire, and get you labeled as a "drug-seeking" patient. Try all of the other types of medications your doctor suggests. If they don't work, then ask if there is anything else you can try. If the doctor says no, don't argue; instead start looking for a second opinion. When you see a new doctor, bring a list of all the medications you've already tried and what effect they had on you.

Unfortunately none of these medications are a cure for chronic pain. All they can do is improve the quality of your life and increase your functionality. While working with your doctor to discover the best combination of medications for your situation, keep the quality of life issue in mind.

If a drug stops your pain but makes it so you cannot do anything but lay in front of the television, then it may not be worth taking on a daily basis. That particular medication may be useful once in a while when the pain is so bad you are already bed-ridden. On other days, use only the drugs that make your pain tolerable enough to get out of the house to run errands, socialize or work.

All medications have side effects. Your pharmacist can give you more information about the particular medication you are taking. A common side effect is weight changes, so it's a good idea to invest in a scale. Gaining three or four pounds a month can add up quickly, and with chronic pain it's very difficult to lose excess weight. Talk to your doctor right away if you start to gain or lose weight after starting a new medication; there may be something equally effective that doesn't affect your metabolism so dramatically.

Probably the most common side effect from pain medication is constipation. A few supplements can help alleviate this problem: Colace stool softener (the generic, docusate sodium, is less expensive and equally effective), flax seed oil, and magnesium. Be sure to drink plenty of water, as dehydration can be a major component with constipation. The stool softener, as the name suggests, makes the waste softer. The flax seed oil will lubricate your system, and magnesium will help get things moving. If you find things are moving too quickly or have become too soft, calcium can help bind and slow the waste down. As you experiment to find the exact dosage of each supplement to work with your body, keep in mind that it may take a few days to feel the effects.

If you feel you need a laxative, taking extra magnesium can be gentler on the system than a stimulant laxative like bisacodyl but may not work as well. Also, external heat (like a heating pad) to your abdomen will slow digestion, while internal heat (like a cup of hot water or tea) will speed things up.

There are many other supplements, herbs, and homeopathic remedies available for various conditions. Take the time to research your options, and then discuss them with your doctor or other qualified practitioner before adding any drugs to your treatment plan.

Keep a list of all the medications (including supplements and herbs) you take with you at all times. If you are ever in an accident or need to go to the emergency room, this information could be vital to your care. Also be sure to tell your pharmacist and all of your doctors every medication you use, so they can alert you to any potential interactions.

As you try different medications, be aware of how they are affecting you both mentally and physically. Also pay attention to how your medications interact. Some may work better together; and some may not work together at all. When using a medication (or dietary supplement) for the first time, take it separately from all of your other drugs. This is so you know if any reaction you have is from the new pill, and not from an interaction with something else. Find a pharmacist you trust, and utilize their knowledge to gain the most from your medications. Even if you have tried every medication available, check with your doctor at least once a year, since new ones are constantly being developed.

Take Action!

❖ Create a list of all the medication you take, and keep it in your wallet. This information will be important if you are ever in an accident or unexpectedly need medical care.

❖ Keep a separate list of all the medications you have tried in the past. Note the name of the drug, when you started and stopped taking it, and why you stopped. This will help you remember what you've already tried in the past to manage your pain.

❖ If you don't remember what you've already tried, your pharmacy can print a list of the prescriptions you've had filled.

Building Your Health Care Team

You are the project manager for your health care. This is a tough role to fill when you don't feel well; however you are the best person for the job. Many people blindly hand off their healthcare to their primary doctor. For a temporary problem, this may work. When you have a chronic issue, you will need to take a more active role in order to get the best care possible. Unless you can afford to keep a doctor on your personal payroll full-time, you are competing with others for the doctor's time and attention. It's not fair; it's just the way it is.

The fact your doctor treats other patients actually benefits you. The doctor learns what helps and what doesn't by working with a larger group of people. When you have an unusual symptom, there's a greater chance the doctor has seen it before in someone else. Remember, they call it "practicing" medicine. Doctors are constantly learning from both the most recent research and their patients.

This may sound obvious, but it's not to everyone: allow only doctors you trust to treat you. A medical degree from a great school does not make someone a good doctor. Your Aunt Bertha may have loved her doctor, but if he gives you the creeps, then go to someone else. Everyone is unique, and this means we communicate in different ways, and our comfort level changes around different people. If you become extremely anxious around your doctor, he will probably dismiss your physical symptoms and send you to a psychiatrist. Then every doctor you see afterwards will read in your medical record about your anxiety issues. Unfortunately, many doctors believe the medical records over the word of the patient sitting in front of them. I've found it's better to change doctors than to subject myself to the unnecessary stress of dealing with someone I don't fully trust. I saw nearly all of the doctors in the Rheumatology department before I met the doctor with whom I trust my health care.

If you have an HMO, they will probably require you to select a primary care physician to manage all the referrals you may need to see specialists. This doctor will have a great deal of control over what other doctors you can consult. Choose carefully. Pay attention to not only the doctor, but also to the doctor's staff. I have stopped seeing doctors because of their receptionist's bad behavior. When I need to see the doctor, I expect to be treated with respect. If I leave a message for the doctor, I expect the doctor to get the correct message within a reasonable amount of time. Remember, it's the medical assistants and secretaries who process all of the paperwork, including referrals and insurance information. Of course, always treat them with respect, no matter how horrible you feel. They are dealing with people in pain and distress all day, every day.

When you have a chronic illness and an HMO, consider what specialists you may need to see before selecting your primary care physician. HMO's often cluster doctors and specialists into medical groups. If your primary care physician is in one group and the specialist you want to see is in another, your HMO will not pay for your visit to the specialist. You are allowed to change physicians and medical groups, however you may need to wait a month for it to become effective. Also, read your plan benefits carefully; some insurance companies have added clauses to restrict the number of times you can change doctors during the year.

Building a relationship with a single doctor is important. This allows the doctor to become familiar with your history and how you describe your symptoms. He or she will know what is considered "normal" for you. Your doctor will be able to quickly read his or her own notes about your case and know what you have already tried for treatment.

Ideally, all of your doctors would communicate with each other about your case and develop a comprehensive treatment plan to help you gain as much improvement as possible. In reality, this rarely happens. You are the contact between doctors. It's up to you to fill in all of your care providers with the relevant details from the others. They may send reports to each other, but that doesn't mean each doctor reads the reports thoroughly. Some do, but not all. It's also a good idea to obtain copies of their reports so you can review them for accuracy.

If you are seeing a physical therapist and you are not responding well, don't expect your doctor to figure it out from a report. You will need to tell him or her yourself. The same is true with the medication you take. Always bring a complete list of everything you take, no matter who prescribed it, including supplements and herbs. Consider making lists of your care providers and the treatments they recommend. If your physical therapist asks you to do some stretches at home, and then your chiropractor recommends different stretches, make sure they know what the other is proposing. It may not benefit you to do both; perhaps you'll need to alternate the days you do the specific stretches so you don't wear yourself out, or you may have to try one for a while and then try the other to see which one helps more.

On your health care team, here are some of the players you'll want working with you:

- Primary Care Doctor – If you're lucky, your primary care doctor will take care of all of your needs. For most people, however, you'll see the primary care doctor when something new or unrelated comes up.

- Specialist – Your Rheumatologist or Neurologist (or whatever fits your case the best) will be your treating physician, and the one from whom you get your prescriptions.

- Psychologist – Living in chronic pain is extremely difficult, and having a trained professional to talk to about your struggles helps immensely. You don't need to be depressed to see a psychologist. A psychologist experienced in dealing with chronic pain patients is an important part of routine care.

- Pharmacist – Insurance companies may offer discounts if you use a preferred mail-order pharmacy, and this is great for medications you have been taking for a long time. While you are experimenting, a good local pharmacy is important. A pharmacist is a specialist in all medications, and they can help you avoid potentially serious problems when taking more than one medication. In addition, they can provide information about what to expect when you start or stop a medication. Most are happy to answer questions either in person or over the phone.

- Physical Therapist – A physical therapist can help you get moving in whatever way your body is capable, and help you develop an exercise routine to do at home.

- Alternative Care practitioners – See the section on Body Work for a detailed list of health care workers who help millions of people living in chronic pain every day.

Being the project manager for your health care is not an easy job. However, no one else can do it as well as you can. You know your body best, so trust yourself. Keep your own notebook for medical visits so you don't have to rely on your memory. Be open to the advice given by professionals, and keep in mind your goal: to have your body and mind functioning at the highest level possible.

Terminal Sentence

I have no time to do things that do not bring joy.
The constant pain of this physical frame
does not mean I must suffer.
Enlightenment is at hand;
all I need to do is open to It and let go.
It is through this disease I am learning body awareness.
When to eat, when to sleep, when to exercise, when to rest.
This disease cannot stop me from doing what I truly love.

I don't know which is worse: being told you have only a year to live, or being told you can expect to live another 30 or 40 years in severe, constant pain. When I was diagnosed with Fibromyalgia, the doctor told me I should not be upset because my body would live just as long as someone with Rheumatoid Arthritis. He didn't understand how intense the pain and weakness had become for me...or that I simply could not accept a diagnosis with no treatment and no cure. I left his office depressed and desperate. When I got home and began researching my new diagnosis, confusion overwhelmed me as I realized I had symptoms that did not fit on the list. In the midst of my internal freak out, I wondered: if these other symptoms were from a terminal illness, would I want to know?

As a Buddhist, I learned about reincarnation and how we move from one body to the next over the course of many lifetimes. I read about the Tibetan masters who used their death as a teaching tool. The master would tell their senior students where and when he would next be born. When a child was identified as a possible reincarnation of the master, the child would be tested by being asked to make a selection from a variety of items brought by the monks. The child would then select the item belonging to the master in his previous life, and return to the monastery to continue his spiritual work. After years of my own practice, I began to have moments of remembrance as pieces of my own past lives reactivated in my awareness. I cannot prove it to anyone, but I know I have had other bodies before this one, and I will have another available to me when this one dies.

Knowing this does not lessen the sting of loss when I think of leaving this world, or when I've said goodbye to others departing for their next journey. Even though I cannot tell you exactly where or when my next incarnation will be, knowing life continues in this and other worlds removes the fear of that transition.

Once we step outside of fear, we can use the knowledge of our own mortality to live better today. Mystics have long used death as an advisor. Framing every action in the context of "what if this were my last act?" changes everything. Taking this powerful stance leaves no room for self-pity, regret, anger or hate. It allows us to consciously focus our energies on what is truly important to us.

The tricky part is we don't know the exact moment of our death. Even when confronted with a terminal illness, doctors can offer only estimates. And even then, anything is possible. An accident could kill the patient while leaving the doctor's office. Or a miracle cure could be discovered and suddenly the terminal illness is no longer terminal. Finding the balance between planning for a realistic future and doing what you love today is key. The best advice my teacher gave me on this point is: Be prepared for the worst, hope for the best, and expect nothing.

Once we realize we don't know when the body will die, we can greet every day as a precious gift because we're not sure if we'll get another one tomorrow. And at the same time, we can dream what we would like to do tomorrow because there is a chance we'll be here. In either case, accepting the body's inevitable end teaches us all we have with any certainty is this moment, right now.

Everyone faces the mortality of the body eventually. Most people seem to prefer to ignore their impending death, feeling it somehow won't happen to them. The truth is death makes us and every other living thing equal. No matter how wonderful or horrible you have been, no matter what you have accomplished or didn't, in the end we all face the same door. The only difference is some are dragged through filled with denial and resistance while others step through with their eyes wide open to the wonder waiting on the other side.

The way we walk through the door of death and into the next life is determined by the sum total of our awareness. Every moment we have the choice to shut down or open up to all the different layers of experience. The more we can open, the greater our awareness becomes, and the wider our view of existence. As we move higher and higher, our suffering diminishes. Just as cars shrink when viewed from an airplane, we see how small our pain is compared to Eternity.

Through the twin practices of meditation and mindfulness we expand our awareness. We use everything in our life as an opportunity to practice. Sometimes we find ourselves stuck on the roller coaster of duality. We rise up, we go down, we twist, and we turn. Sometimes we scream; other times we laugh in sheer delight. In our terror, we wish for it to end; then we realize that it will in fact end – and that causes even more terror. In our laughter, we feel only the exhilaration of the moment.

Whether we are in terror or joy, we can stand back and watch ourselves on the roller coaster. By standing firmly in the present moment, we can see the mind's reaction to the circumstances of life and the impending death of the body. We can witness all the different games the mind plays as it moves through each twist and turn and dip. From this place of silence, we realize we are not the mind and we are not the body. At that moment, no matter what is happening to or around us, we are free.

Mystery Of The Month

The fourth or fifth time I went to my doctor complaining of fatigue, pain, and flu-like symptoms, he called me his "mystery of the month" because he didn't understand why I kept getting sick. My blood tests were essentially normal – there were a few irregularities, but nothing to explain why I would feel so weak and then be fine a short time later. He prescribed antibiotics during the first few visits, which helped while I took them. Then in a few weeks, the mysterious illness would return, and I would find myself literally stuck on the floor unable to get up.

He sent me off to a specialist, who sent me to another specialist, and thus my odyssey through the health care system began. I explored medical doctors and complementary health care practitioners. Because my tests didn't reveal the cause of my body issues, I was sent to a psychiatrist. The psychiatrist sent me back to the medical doctors. Fourteen practitioners later, I finally got a diagnosis of Fibromyalgia and Temporomandibular Joint Dysfunction (TMD).

The more I read about it, the less certain I felt. Another doctor said I also had Chronic Fatigue Syndrome, and yet another one told me the trigger points in my muscles were the result of a disease called Chronic Myofascial Pain. The common themes of these illnesses soon became apparent: they cannot be diagnosed with a blood test, they will not kill you, once fully developed the symptoms remain fairly stable, and they can be managed with what the doctors like to call lifestyle changes.

I continued to search for information about these illnesses and found that while medical science makes amazing discoveries every day, many questions remain unanswered. There are millions of people with various diseases waiting for a cure or at least a treatment that works. Among these are people like me who have been diagnosed with TMD, Chronic Fatigue Syndrome, Fibromyalgia, and Chronic Myofascial Pain.

Some doctors have diagnosed me with all four of these medical conditions as separate maladies, while other doctors use the last three terms interchangeably and consider TMD a common complication of them. Since the current treatments are similar for all three conditions, doctors will probably continue to use the different names to describe the same set of symptoms. Which term they use typically depends upon their specialty. A Rheumatologist is more likely to give a diagnosis of Fibromyalgia, while an Internal Medicine doctor may call it Chronic Fatigue Syndrome or Chronic Myofascial Pain. Some doctors will say the patient with predominant pain has Fibromyalgia, while the patient with predominant fatigue complaints will be labeled with Chronic Fatigue Syndrome. Unless the doctor is involved with research, it probably doesn't matter all that much what they call the illness. The important thing is if they can help the patient.

Based on my own research, I have come to believe there are some significant differences in these conditions. The primary difference between Chronic

Fatigue Syndrome and Fibromyalgia seems to be in how the illness first presents itself. Chronic Myofascial Pain, on the other hand, appears to be an entirely separate disease often found in patients with TMD, Fibromyalgia and/or Chronic Fatigue Syndrome, as well as with many types of Arthritis.

The only common thread I found through most of the research was that these illnesses were deemed to not be progressive. Progressive means the disease causes the patient to deteriorate over time despite rest and treatment. This discovery disturbed me, since my body continued to deteriorate even with proper lifestyle changes and treatment. When new symptoms involving trouble breathing and severe lightheadedness reached the point where I could no longer ignore them, I returned to my doctors for an explanation. My primary care doctor and most of the specialists I saw told me: "It must be the Fibromyalgia." My Rheumatologist disagreed, but didn't have any answers for me. She encouraged me to keep looking for the cause, thinking there must be something else going on in my body.

I began my search over again with a new set of doctors, and eventually found a clinic specializing in difficult to diagnose conditions. The initial tests showed I was positive for Toxoplasmosis and active Epstein-Barr virus, which indicated a compromised immune system. My symptoms met the diagnostic criteria for Lyme disease and its many co-infections, and the blood tests provided an indirect confirmation. The loopy feeling of lightheadedness went away after being treated for Toxoplasmosis, for which I am grateful. I went on intense antibiotic treatment for a year, but most of my symptoms continue to persist. Since the antibiotic treatment did not improve my functionality and it had unwanted gastro-intestinal side effects, I decided to discontinue it and look for other options. Fortunately, I am stubborn and have a strong mind – even though it doesn't always work correctly – so I will continue to learn and grow spiritually with my "mystery of the month" diagnosis. In practical terms, I will keep working towards greater functionality as I discover how to operate this ever-changing body at maximum efficiency. Every day is a new adventure.

Below I provide a brief synopsis of the five conditions doctors have labeled me with, as I understand them. Entire books have been written about each of these illnesses, many of them offering different theories and treatments. The research continues daily, as scientists strive to understand the details of these conditions and how best to correct them. The following is intended to provide a basic understanding of these illnesses in order to direct you towards your own research and treatment options, should you choose to do so.

Chronic Fatigue Syndrome (CFS)

Chronic Fatigue Syndrome (CFS) is a diagnosis of exclusion because there is no blood test, brain scan or other lab test to diagnose it. The primary complaint is persistent, unexplained fatigue that doesn't get better with rest. The fatigue also results in a significant reduction in your previous level of activity. In addition to the fatigue, people with CFS also experience (for over six months) at least four of the following symptoms: impaired memory or concentration; extreme, prolonged exhaustion and sickness following physical or mental activity; un-refreshing sleep; muscle pain; multi-joint pain without swelling or redness; headaches of a new type or severity; frequent or recurring sore throat; tender lymph nodes.

When you visit your doctor, he or she will go through your history to review any medications and any other possible causes for how you feel. The doctor should also perform a thorough physical and mental examination before ordering a series of tests to check for other illnesses. The symptoms of Chronic Fatigue Syndrome are similar to many other illnesses including mononucleosis, Lyme disease, lupus, multiple sclerosis, fibromyalgia, primary sleep disorders, severe obesity and major depressive disorders. Medications can also cause side effects similar to the symptoms of CFS.

Because CFS can resemble many other disorders, it's important not to self-diagnose CFS. It's not uncommon for people to mistakenly assume they have chronic fatigue syndrome when they have another illness that needs to be treated. If you have CFS symptoms, consult a health care professional to determine if any other conditions are responsible for your symptoms. A CFS diagnosis can be made only after other conditions have been excluded.

It's also important not to delay seeking a diagnosis and medical care. CDC research suggests that early diagnosis and treatment of CFS can increase the likelihood of improvement.

(Information from: http://www.cdc.gov/cfs/cfsdiagnosis.htm)

Fibromyalgia (FM)

The hallmark of Fibromyalgia is the unpredictable flares of pain. They can last for minutes, hours, or months. Sometimes you can pinpoint a cause, like lifting something too heavy or standing too long. Other times the flare begins for no apparent reason. When in a flare, it feels as if every nerve ending in the body has been activated by pain signals. It may feel like you suddenly have a nasty bruise, though there is no discoloration on the skin. Even the slightest touch or hug from a well-meaning friend feels like being bludgeoned. There are not enough painkillers in the world to completely eradicate the pain of a Fibromyalgia flare. Rest, warm baths, hot packs, and time seem to be the only things that eventually provide a small amount of relief. Really, the only things one can do are: wait it out and do everything possible not to exacerbate it. This means resting and very gentle stretching every couple of hours. Distracting the mind from the pain can make this waiting game more tolerable.

Fibromyalgia often is lumped into the Arthritis category and is mainly treated by Rheumatologists, since it primarily affects the soft tissue of the body. Often the patients describe their pain being in the joints when it is actually the soft tissue attached to the joint causing the pain. Current research is pointing towards a problem with the autonomic nervous system and how it works with the muscles, nerves, and pain receptors.

There has been much debate about the symptoms involved with Fibromyalgia; however, after many years of research, a set of diagnostic criteria evolved. In

February 1990, the American College of Rheumatology published a study in which researchers were able to determine which patients had Fibromyalgia from a set of control patients who had other diseases with similar pain symptoms. They accomplished this through the use of a Tender Point Exam. They discovered people with Fibromyalgia had pain (not just tenderness) when specific points on the body were pressed with light pressure. The published study containing the criteria can be found at:

http://www.rheumatology.org/publications/classification/
fibromyalgia/1990_Criteria_for_Classification_Fibro.asp

The researchers concluded a diagnosis of Fibromyalgia should be made for patients with both widespread pain (above and below the waist on both sides) and at least 11 out of 18 specific tender points that are painful upon palpitation.

They also discovered that many, but not all, patients with Fibromyalgia experience fatigue, sleep disturbances (waking un-refreshed), and muscle stiffness. Other symptoms now associated with Fibromyalgia also include: irritable bowel syndrome, painful menstrual periods, urinary urgency and interstitial cystitis, hypersensitivity to touch, light, sound and chemicals, chronic headaches, jaw pain and TMJ disorder, numbness and tingling sensations, dizziness, and cognitive or memory impairment.

The cognitive problems are typically called "Fibrofog" by patients because it feels as if your mind is muddled. The Fibrofog comes and goes. One minute it may be difficult to understand what people are saying, or you may forget simple words when talking, while in another case you may forget how to get somewhere that you've been to many times before. It occurs more frequently when you have exhausted yourself by doing too much and during flares of high pain. Fibrofog also occurs without warning, and goes away just as quickly.

Fibromyalgia may be present with other diseases, so your doctor should rule out any other conditions with similar symptoms. After diagnosis, it's also important to keep your doctor from labeling every new symptom as part of Fibromyalgia. If another condition is present, there may be a treatment for it, which may help reduce the severity of the Fibromyalgia symptoms.

If you believe you may have Fibromyalgia, plan to rest after your doctor's appointment. The Tender Point Exam, while helpful in diagnosing the illness, can cause increased pain for a prolonged period of time at the tender point sites.

Chronic Myofascial Pain (CMP)

Chronic Myofascial Pain (CMP) is a disease characterized by an abnormality in the muscle tissue, which makes the muscles prone to developing trigger points. A trigger point is a knot in the fibers of the muscle, and can typically be felt by a massage therapist or other trained body worker. Trigger points often refer pain to other parts of the body and can cause a variety of non-muscle symptoms. For example, a trigger point in a neck muscle can cause headaches, dizziness, and vision problems. A trigger point in the upper shoulder can cause pain down the arm. If a nerve is entangled in the trigger point, you may also experience numbness and tingling. Some trigger points are active, where you feel the pain all the time or when you use the affected muscle. Other trigger points are latent, where they cause pain only when pressure is applied.

With Chronic Myofascial Pain, trigger points have been created in multiple muscles. This occurs because the first trigger point pulls the fibers of the muscle tight, and causes a strain on the adjacent muscles. Left untreated, the original trigger point becomes tighter and tighter, putting more and more strain on the adjacent muscles. This causes another trigger point to be created in each of those muscles. The process continues until the entire body is riddled with trigger points.

While trigger points are common in the general population, the tendency to develop trigger points in the adjacent muscles is not. Something in the muscles of people with CMP causes a rapid development of trigger points from one muscle to the next. A simple shoulder strain can develop into widespread debilitating pain in a matter of months as trigger points form in the arm, neck and back muscles.

The good news is CMP can be successfully treated. The bad news for people with Fibromyalgia and Chronic Fatigue Syndrome is the treatment for CMP usually exacerbates Fibromyalgia and CFS symptoms, making the treatment intolerable. The two most common treatments for trigger points are a spray and stretch technique performed by a trained physical therapist, or trigger point release performed by a trained massage therapist using a deep tissue technique. Both techniques involve manually rubbing across the trigger point to release the tangled muscle fibers. Each trigger point can take several sessions to release.

The hypersensitivity of most Fibromyalgia patients makes this treatment a torture session and is impractical because of the long flare of pain it typically causes. In addition to the increased pain, the muscles themselves tend to become contracted after a session and prevent the trigger point from releasing completely. For people with Chronic Fatigue Syndrome, the treatment can be problematic because their bodies do not recover well from physical stress due to the lack of restorative sleep. In short, the treatment becomes worse than the disease for most people with FM and CFS because of this rebound effect.

For people who can tolerate the treatment, immense relief can be gained by releasing trigger points. To keep the trigger points from reforming, a program of stretching, self-massage, and light exercise is essential.

Learning about trigger points can be useful in uncovering the cause of mysterious symptoms. The best book I've found is *The Trigger Point Therapy Workbook: Your Self-Treatment Guide for Pain Relief* by Clair Davies. Even if you cannot tolerate the full treatment, you may find some relief by doing self-treatment on your most painful trigger points.

Temporomandibular Joint Dysfunction (TMD)

If you have facial pain, ear pain, a sore neck, dizziness, or vision problems, it could be related to your temporomandibular joint. The TMJ, or jaw joint, is the most complex joint within the body. It actually consists of two joints, one on each side of the face, that work together to move up and down, forwards and backwards, and side to side. This powerful and beautifully designed work of art allows us to both feed ourselves and to express ourselves through speech and facial expressions. Surrounded by muscles and nerves, the jaw joint can bring us to our knees when it malfunctions. Without our being conscious of it, the distortions it can cause to our facial muscles can sour our mood, and it can insidiously make us not want to eat or talk. Opening the mouth to scream often makes it worse.

Adding to the horror of pain and the frightening sensation of your mouth stuck or of the sound of pops and clicks, is the fact that there is not one medical profession that specializes in treating diseases of the temporomandibular joint. There are many types of doctors who treat TMD, but there is not a specialty dedicated just to this very special set of joints. During your adventure to discover a treatment that works for you, you may consult an Oral Surgeon, a Neurologist, a Rheumatologist, a physical therapist, and a pain specialist.

At a routine cleaning, my dentist noticed my jaw opening was crooked. This discovery started me on a path to discover the cause of my debilitating headaches and ear pain. After consulting my insurance booklet, I learned my dental insurance would not cover treatment of the TMJ, but my health insurance would. (The fuzzy area of whether it's a tooth problem or a face problem is the root of many insurance nightmares for TMD patients.) My primary care doctor sent me to an Ear-Nose-

Throat specialist, who then sent me to an Oral Surgeon. The Oral Surgeon appeared to be a specialist; however I learned the hard way he was not. The treatments he prescribed all made the pain and dysfunction worse. The good news is the experience taught me to trust myself and advocate for my health care.

Because so little is known about the causes of TMJ problems, it is challenging to find solutions. This complex joint includes muscles, nerves, tendons, and a disc between the two bones. If any small part of the package becomes misaligned or irritated, it can cause TMD. Muscles can become tight enough to pull one side out of alignment and cause the teeth not to fit together properly when chewing. If the dentist files down the teeth to make them fit, and then the muscle relaxes, the pain and dysfunction will start up all over again. The same is true of any surgical options. Therefore, the best treatments to explore involve non-permanent alterations.

There are no treatments that work for everyone. I was told to completely rest my jaw for two weeks and eat only liquid food. This made everything tighter and increased the pain. Then I was given a custom-made mouth splint with the promise it would relax my jaw muscles and told to wear it all day and all night, except when eating. When I complained that the splint made the pain worse, I was told it simply needed to be adjusted and I needed to be patient and let it work. After two months, I was completely incapacitated by the pain.

Current recommendations from The TMJ Association (www.TMJ.org) stipulate that if patients try a mouth splint it should be used for only short periods of time initially and if any discomfort occurs, it should be discontinued immediately because in many cases a mouth splint can make the condition worsen.

Fortunately, I eventually found a chiropractor who is able to do a gentle adjustment to my jaw and push it back into place. Yawning, flossing my teeth, or even laughing is enough to knock the jaw joint out again. For me, I look at the treatment as part of my body's regular maintenance.

The most helpful home treatments I've found are icepacks on my jaw and a hot pack on my neck. For medication, an anti-inflammatory pill helps with my jaw and other muscles, and a topical cream (Ketoprofen 10% cream) made at a compounding pharmacy also helps keep the face swelling down.

Being mindful of the food I eat is also an important part of daily care. Obviously I no longer chew gum, and I limit hard, crunchy food. Crunching activates pleasure centers in the brain, so I haven't given up all crunchy things, but I do look for softer options; for example I'll choose the Pop-Chips brand potato chips instead of the Kettle-Cooked brand, and I'll cook my carrots instead of eating them raw. Too much laughing and smiling can also irritate my jaw, but there's no way I'll give that up!

The latest research is looking at connections between TMD, CMP, Chronic Fatigue Syndrome, Fibromyalgia, and Endometriosis as they are finding these conditions often occur together. If you are affected by TMD, first off, know that you are not alone and people are looking for solutions. While it may be difficult, take your time in evaluating your options. Choose reversible treatments over permanent ones, and ask lots and lots of questions before undergoing any procedures. Experiment and trust your own experiences of what works for you.

Lyme Disease and Co-infections

Lyme disease and its associated co-infections affect multiple body systems and many of the symptoms are similar to both Fibromyalgia and Chronic Fatigue Syndrome. There may be excessive fatigue, pain in the muscles and joints, and cognitive problems. Left untreated, Lyme can affect the central nervous system, the heart, and damage the immune system causing a variety of severe problems.

Many Lyme patients describe the onset of the disease as a sudden flu-like illness that lasts for a week or two, goes away, and then returns. Lyme disease is transmitted by tick bites, and is often accompanied by other infections from the same tick. Each bacteria and parasite causing the infections is unique and may require different antibiotic treatments.

Years ago it was thought Lyme disease only occurs in certain parts of the country; new research suggests it can be acquired anywhere. Many people with Lyme disease do not remember ever being bit by a tick. Of those who do remember being bitten, only a small percentage get the bulls-eye rash associated with Lyme.

Doctors who specialize in researching and treating Lyme disease and its associated co-infections have determined that Lyme disease is a clinical diagnosis, based on the signs and symptoms of the patient. According to ILADS (International Lyme and Associated

Disease Society), the initial screening test recommended by the CDC misses 35% of culture proven Lyme disease and therefore is unacceptable as a first-step screening test. They also note that antibody titers appear to decline over time, so the second step test, the Western Blot, may not be able to detect the disease in people who have had it for a long time.

The CDC on the other hand, insists the screening test is "very sensitive, meaning that almost everyone with Lyme disease, and some people who don't have Lyme disease, will test positive." They do caution that in the very early stages of the disease, the test may come back as a false-negative, and should not be used to rule out Lyme disease as a possible diagnosis.

In addition to the disagreement over the accuracy of the blood tests, there is also much debate over the treatment of Lyme disease. Some doctors feel the only treatment is a short course of antibiotics, and patients who do not respond must have something else wrong. Other doctors have had success by treating patients with long-term antibiotic therapy. Doctors and researchers will mostly likely continue to argue the issues for many more years.

If your illness continues to progress despite treatment and proper self-care, you need to return to your doctor. Once everything else has been ruled out, you may want to investigate the possibility of having Lyme disease if there is any chance you could have been bitten by a tick.

Because of the controversy, you may want to search for an expert in your area. By searching the Internet for "Lyme disease doctors" you should be able to find websites that will help connect you with doctors who specialize in Lyme disease. When making an appointment with the local doctor, always ask if the doctor still treats people with Lyme disease. Because of the amount of contradictory research, some doctors may choose to no longer specialize in treating this disease.

Be persistent as you seek help for your illness, no matter what it is, and don't be afraid to ask for a second opinion. You know your body the best.

Tips For Pain Flares

We meditate, we practice mindfulness, we pace ourselves – and yet, sometimes we still find ourselves in a severe flare of pain. For many of us, the first instinct is to push through it. Our thinking becomes muddled by pain, and we forget about pacing. Next to go is our practice of mindfulness, and we find ourselves frustrated and depressed. And in this state, it's difficult to remember meditation is the way out of suffering.

Here is a list of tips to deal with severe pain flares. These are all things to do at home, because it's not every day we can get to our favorite body worker. And even when we do see the chiropractor or acupuncturist or massage therapist, it's easy to undo their work. Try these tips and see what works for you.

- Treat your body like a sacred object. After all, it is a manifestation of God.

- Meditate every day. Even a few minutes of meditation can boost your energy and improve your mood. When you don't feel like sitting is often the time you need it the most.

- Maintain your mind through the practice of mindfulness. Pay attention to your thoughts and constantly direct them to higher and happier states of mind, no matter what is happening to or around you. Focus on beauty and gratitude to pull you up, and strive to see the positive side of every situation you encounter.

- Practice pacing and be mindful of your body at all times. If an action you are performing (or a position you are sitting or lying in) is increasing your pain, make the appropriate adjustments. If you cannot do it differently, then take a break until the pain recedes. An example: You're putting three plates in the cabinet at a time and your pain is increasing. Start putting just one plate away at a time. It may take longer, but you'll be in less pain when you're done.

- Remember pain is a transitory sensation. Sometimes it feels like it will last forever, feeling exactly the same. However, even chronic pain has variations, although they may be slight. We can watch for these variations to remind ourselves of pain's transitory nature.

- Distract yourself from the sensation by concentrating on a different sensation. It may be a sound, a video, or the texture of a soft blanket that gives you a momentary break from the feeling of pain.

- Heat up a hot pack, or put on a cold pack. If you feel heat coming from your muscles, the cold pack will most likely work the best. If your muscles feel unbearably tight, try the hot pack. You can also try alternating them every twenty minutes to help get the circulation going. When the whole body is in spasm, hot packs on your lower back and neck can calm things down.

- Stretch like a cat. Cats stretch every time they get up. Even if they jump up in fright, once the threat is gone, they stop and stretch. There's no regimented way to stretch; do whatever feels good at the moment, giving all of your muscles the opportunity to lengthen before moving around, before settling into bed for the night, and during long rests on the couch. Remember, a stretch is never painful; rather, it is a gentle pulling sensation.

- My favorite stretch for a sore neck and shoulders: Put pillows on a table and pull up a chair. Rest your head on the pillows, allowing your arms to hang loosely by your side. Adjust the height of the pillows or chair to achieve a relaxing passive stretch.

- Roll your ankles in small circles, first in one direction, then the other. Roll your shoulders gently, one at a time. Roll your neck. Be aware of any resistance as you roll; if it hurts, try rolling the opposite direction or change the size of the circle. Never force a movement; if your body doesn't want to roll that way, it's OK. Do only a few rolls at a time.

- Use a Theracane self-massage tool daily. This tool looks like a long hook with a variety of knobs, which allows you to massage your entire body with minimal strain. It costs around $40 and comes with an instruction book.

- Take lots of breaks. While you are resting, DO NOTHING. Reading a book or magazine takes energy and uses your brain, arms and hands, which means reading is not resting. If you need something to keep your mind busy, then watch a video or listen to music.

- If you have one, plug in your TENS unit. The pulsing of the electrodes interrupts the pain signals coming from your muscles. If you don't have one, ask your doctor or chiropractor if one would help your pain.

- Use a pillow on your lap while driving to relive arm and shoulder pain. This is especially helpful on the way home from receiving bodywork at the chiropractor or physical therapist. I keep a u-shaped travel pillow in the car. When I'm driving, I rest my arms on it so I can reach the steering wheel without my shoulders having to hold my arms up. When I'm a passenger, I use the pillow to support my neck.

- Learn to say NO without guilt, sadness, anger, or remorse. You are the only one who knows what your body can tolerate today. Respect your body by declining to do things that increase pain, or by leaving early. Remember to check-in with your body frequently because things can change from hour to hour. You do not need to explain yourself to anyone; if you feel the need to say something before leaving, let your friend know you're tired and need to rest.

- Remember all people have something going on in their life with the potential to cause suffering. While chronic pain is certainly very difficult to live with, others also face challenges every day that intrude on their peace of mind.

- Warm baths help to soothe sore muscles. If you don't have a bathtub, then soak your feet in a large pan or in one of the many foot bath/spa products available. Bath salts vary widely, and I've found some to be more helpful than others. In my experience, pink Himalayan Crystal Salt is the best, but can be hard to find. My next choice is Dead Sea Salt. If you cannot find either of these, then try plain Sea Salt or Epsom Salt. Lavender oil (check to make sure it's real lavender, and not just fragrance) is also helpful, as it has a relaxing effect.

- A spa pillow for the bathtub is helpful. You can also try rolling up a washcloth to provide cushioning for your neck and head in the tub.

- Keep a variety of pillows for your bed and your couch, so you can switch whenever you need to. Placing a pillow between or under your knees can also help relieve pressure points.

- Headphones and a CD or MP3 player with relaxing music on your nightstand will give you something to focus on as you let your body rest during the nights you wake up and cannot fall back asleep.

- Always be positive, optimistic, and realistic.

Tips For Daily Living

This list of tips has been developed through years of practice. They are ways to make our use of energy more efficient. Some may seem commonsense while others are more obscure. Some of these tips have already been presented elsewhere in this book, however I thought it would be helpful to list the most important ones all in one place. Use this collection along with the *Tips for Pain Flares* chapter to build your own efficient life.

♦ It was just listed in the previous chapter, but worth repeating: Practice meditation, mindfulness, and pacing every day.

♦ Balance your life by alternating heavy activity, light activity, and rest. For some people, a heavy activity may be going to the store. A light activity may be reading a book or magazine.

♦ Journal writing provides an outlet for you to vent your frustrations and record your successes, without depending upon anyone else for support. If you have trouble starting the writing process, check out one of the many books available on the subject. Remember, you don't ever need to share your journal; allow yourself to write whatever you want. You can always shred the entries you don't like!

- If you find yourself over-doing on a regular basis, use a portable kitchen timer to remind yourself to take breaks.

- Invest in an electric toothbrush. It not only helps keep your teeth cleaner, it can reduce the hand pain caused by gripping a manual toothbrush.

- Floss daily, or as often as you can. If you have trouble holding the string, use a floss pick. Less plaque and tartar build up means less pain at the dentist, and may even reduce your risk for many other health problems. If flossing makes your gums sore, rinse with warm salt water before and after flossing. Look for a dentist who offers ultrasound cleaning; it's faster and less painful than the pick.

- Find a form of exercise you can do. I have increased pain when I do repetitive motions, which makes it difficult (if not impossible) for me to do most traditional forms of exercise. I discovered a senior citizen's Tai Chi class my body can handle. I cannot do most of the warm-up exercises, so I do as much as I can and then rest. Tai Chi provides enough variety of movement so I don't get worn out as quickly. You don't need to be a senior citizen to join classes designed for them; just let the teacher know you are disabled. Others have found success with gentle yoga classes. I have also begun to use the Nintendo Wii Fit video game, which allows me to exercise at my own level in my home. Explore to find something you enjoy.

◆ Moderation in all things (including moderation!) is key.

◆ Organize. Create files for all the paperwork you need or want to keep. Name files with phrases that make sense to you; ask yourself: "where would I look for this when I need it later?" If you don't have a file cabinet, get one. Also organize your kitchen so the dishes you use most frequently are on the lower shelves and easy to reach.

◆ Handle mail once. If you're not ready to deal with the mail when you bring it in, put it on the table and wait until you are. Then go through the mail and file, toss, or put in an action pile. Take action (for example, pay bills) as soon as possible. Don't create a huge pile of bills to pay later. It takes less energy to write one check a day than it does to write five checks all at once at the end of the week.

◆ Clear out the clutter. A cluttered home can sap your energy. If your home has become cluttered, dedicate ten or twenty minutes per week (or more often if your body allows) to clearing away the clutter. Start with one drawer, one table, or one closet, or one bookcase. Be ruthless – ask yourself if you really intend to read the magazine that's been sitting under the coffee table for a month. By doing a little bit at a time, you'll start to see progress and will be less inclined to let it pile up again.

◆ Hire a cleaning service. Heavy cleaning like scrubbing the shower or mopping the floor is very hard on a person with chronic pain. The energy you save by hiring someone can be put towards organizing and clearing away clutter. Less expensive options are friends or college students who need some extra money. If there is no room in your budget for cleaning help, break up the task into small projects and spread it out over several days.

- Use tools to help with everyday tasks. Keep a pair of pliers in the kitchen to open the safety tab on milk bottles and try a pair of tweezers to open the plastic seal on eye-drops or pill bottles.

- A high-quality electric can-opener is worth the investment if you regularly use canned food. For cans with a pull-tab, use the pliers.

- An easy-grip bottle opener is another kitchen essential.

- If you are strong enough, a pet can be a wonderful friend. Visit your local shelter and ask what exactly is required of you, figure out what you can do, and see if there's a good match for you. Cats can be fairly low-maintenance; however they still need to play, be fed and their litter box cleaned daily, as well as annual check-ups at the vet. A lightweight one-pound kitten grows into a fifteen-pound cat very quickly. Another option is becoming a volunteer at your local shelter, where you can help socialize the dogs or cats while playing.

- Use a date-book and plan activities that are fun for you. Include rest periods in your daily plan. Life can easily become a series of doctor appointments, which can drive anyone towards depression. By using a day planner, you can see how much is on your plate, and when things need to be re-arranged. Be sure to write down all the projects you plan to do, even the small things around the house. The small stuff can add up quickly, leaving you wondering why you don't have the energy to do what you love. Make sure you have at least one or two "want-to's" on your calendar each month, to balance all the "need-to's" you must do.

Taking Refuge

God is with us in our failure as much as in our success.
It is only when we stop trying that we create
the illusion we are separate from God.
God is never separate from us, even when we believe it to be so.

The Buddhist tradition contains a wonderful practice called "Taking Refuge in the Three Jewels." There is a similar practice in Christianity, where practitioners take Christ as their Savior. I suspect most religious traditions share this common theme of taking refuge in something greater than the personal self. When you feel isolated, you can reach for this line into Light, in whatever form is appropriate for you.

The Three Jewels are the Buddha, the Dharma, and the Sangha. The Buddha represents the Enlightened One, a person who has united their mind (and entire being) with God. Buddhas are not God, and are not worshipped. Rather, you could think of a Buddha as one of God's really close friends. A Buddha no longer wants anything from God – he or she is simply present with God in every aspect. Everyone has the potential to be a Buddha; when we take refuge in the Buddha, we accept and recognize this possibility for ourselves.

The Dharma is the highest truth in action. It is the collection of teachings that lead us to experience our full potential. Dharma is the path we follow to wisdom. By taking refuge in the Dharma, we set our intent to find and follow the highest truth we can access.

The Sangha is the community of committed practitioners. They are all the seekers who have gone before us and have fulfilled their highest potential. They are the ones whose lives have become a constant meditation. They are also the ones who are still struggling against the bonds of their attachments, and even though it's difficult, they practice their path every day. Taking refuge in the Sangha reminds us of the success others experienced and that we are not alone on the Path.

The grueling experience of chronic pain can quickly overshadow everything beautiful in this world. No one can fully understand the depth of another person's pain, and this can make you feel disconnected. Taking Refuge is a powerful step beyond suffering.

You don't need to do any special rituals or visit a holy place, although that can be fun and inspiring. You don't need to meet with a teacher or tell your family and friends. It is a private and personal practice of connecting with the Divine present within you. All you need to do is remember.

Some people may do this every day. Others may do it only when they feel lost. It's up to you. Taking Refuge is easy. With your mind focused, say to yourself: I take refuge in the Buddha, the Dharma, and the Sangha. Say it a few times, and spend a few moments contemplating what the Three Jewels mean to you.

Take Action!

❖ Contemplate the meaning of the spiritual symbols that are meaningful to you.

❖ Whenever you are feeling stuck or lost, stop and take refuge in whatever spiritual symbols and traditions are most powerful for you.

The Most Important Moment

"Let the body be preoccupied with illness,
but, O mind, dwell forever in God's Bliss!"
~Ramakrishna

When most people think about their lives, they remember only the big events like birthdays, meeting someone special, weddings, and great vacations. However, our lives are really made up of all the small, seemingly insignificant activities. Eating breakfast in the morning, kissing your spouse before they leave for work, and washing the dishes are all very tiny moments, yet they are the most important. It is during each of these moments we define who we are. As we move through these everyday actions, we create ourselves through our attention.

How aware were you when you washed the dishes? Were you lost in thought, a million miles away? Or were you fully present, doing your best? Do you remember what your breakfast tasted like? Did you enjoy it? Or was it another lost moment?

It's helpful to have something to look forward to, and it's fun to remember past activities that were powerful for us. In the end, though, these big events do not add up to very much. One birthday dinner does not shape us as much as a daily walk to the mailbox.

In our ordinary daily activities, we let loose and see who we really are. There's no need to put on a performance like most people do when they attend a special party. When we throw our freshly washed clothes in a heap on the dresser it shows us how we actually feel: rushed, tired, sore. When we put the clothes away neatly, it once again shows us how we're doing.

Because you live with chronic pain, it's tempting to relive your fond memories in your mind, over and over. After all, there may not be as many of these moments as you would like. Once in a while, it's fun to reminisce. But it doesn't help you grow. And when done excessively, it can make you melancholy.

Instead, strive to live for today. Treat everything you do as if it were the most important thing in the world. Whether it's making your body comfortable on the couch while you rest or buttering your toast, it deserves your full attention.

When you live this way, giving care to the small details of your life, every day becomes special. There's no need to wait for someone to take you out to your favorite restaurant or for a perfect sunset. As you move through these ordinary moments mindfully, your overall level of awareness is revealed. And as you keep your mind in the present you begin to realize this moment, right now, is glorious and beautiful. Every small thing you do with your whole being, you do with love, and as a result you see the wonder, the magic, and mystery of Light.

Making Peace With Pain

If you're like most of us, you read through this book and thought about doing a few of the suggestions. Then you became busy with your life, and you forgot all about them.

Before you put this book back on the shelf, read the book again, and perhaps even a third or fourth time. During these readings, slowly chew on the concepts presented, so they have time to sink into your mind. Do the "Take Action" tasks as you come across them to the best of your ability. There are many layers of information within these pages. Your job as you read is to discover what works for you today.

Once you finish reading the book a few times, keep it nearby for the tough days. When you are struggling, flip it open and practice the lesson or suggestions in whatever chapter you randomly selected. Keep in mind as you practice, some of the techniques may sound simple, but they are by no means easy. Some of them may even offend your ego. I offer no apology; I am merely sharing with you what has worked for me. Despite the obstacles I have faced in the past and the physical challenges I live with today, these teachings have allowed me to create an uncommonly fine life. My wish is they do the same for you.

The first few pages contain a set of Short Instructions intended to help you begin your own journey. Refer back to these first few pages and practice the techniques at least once each day. Continue to do this until meditation and mindfulness become part of your daily life.

I have succeeded on this path not because of who I am, but because of what I have become: a warrior.

When we think of warriors, we often picture violence. You may think you are at war with your body, but you are not. Your body is merely a vehicle. Would you go to war with your car if it broke down on the side of the road? Or would you do whatever you could to get it running again?

We all have a warrior spirit within us. Most people experience it only in connection with righteous anger. We can intentionally access this powerful part of us, and use it whenever we need that extra rush of energy. A warrior commits to action that will serve her cause. If you want to be at peace with pain, it will take practice and dedication. It will force you to decide between anger and love.

Peace doesn't mean everything works out the way we want it to, nor does it mean to be apathetic. Inner peace comes from the recognition that we are more than these fragile bodies. It comes from connecting with everyone and everything on a level deeper than the sensorial world. Simply put, it comes from love. And we discover this profound love through meditation.

We use the warrior part of our being to call ourselves on our own indulgences. We know when we're wallowing in self-pity or stewing in anger. Our warrior-self will pull us out, without punishment, and get us to practice mindfulness and sit in meditation each day. It's the fierce part of us that says "enough" and lets go of the anger, the sorrow, and the hate. The warrior is what allows us to focus on Light and make peace with pain.

Each day we can cultivate the warrior within through the practices of meditation and mindfulness. Once the mind is open, we can sit like a child in wonder and awe of all that life is. When we begin to fall, the warrior is there, always ready to pull us back on track.

Deeper Still

When every nerve in my body fires in pain
And every muscle fiber contracts in spasm
I want to scream and let hot tears flood from my eyes
But the crying and screaming only intensifies the spasms of pain.
I learned instead to dive deep.

Deep below the turbulent waves of this fragile body,
Deep beyond the anger, the fear, the sorrow of pain,
Deep beneath the rationality of everything I think I know
I melt into the still point within.

In the silence the light burns brighter than ten-thousand suns.
At the edge of awareness, I feel the torment of the body's pain.
I see the agony of emotional despair.
I hear the frustration of the mind
Grasping to control the crashing waves.
None of it matters to me as
I melt into the still point within.

Here, in the silence, I know I am not this fragile body.
I taste the sweetness of unconditional joy;
A smile erupts under my lips.

Deeper still, this thing called I dissolves.
There is only perfect peace
Shining brighter than ten-thousand suns,
Burning its very essence
To Light all the worlds.

Resources

The following lists are a short sample of the resources that have helped me develop the highest quality life possible. Browse through them and see what may help you. Keep your own list of favorites to make it easy for you to find inspiration when you need it most.

Books

Books are wonderful doorways. They teach and inspire and carry us into new worlds. Not only do we learn the author's message, we also learn about ourselves each time we react to a message. I have way too many favorites to include them all, so here are the ones I think you may enjoy the most.

When Things Fall Apart: Heart Advice for Difficult Times
Pema Chodron

Finding a Joyful Life in the Heart of Pain
Darlene Cohen

Total Relaxation - The Complete Program to Overcome Stress, Tension, Worry and Fatigue
Dr. Frederick Lenz

The Trigger Point Therapy Workbook: Your Self-Treatment Guide for Pain Relief
Clair Davies

Fibromyalgia and Chronic Myofascial Pain: A Survival Manual
Devin J. Starlanyl and Mary Ellen Copeland

Your Perfect Right: Assertiveness and Equality in Your Life and Relationships
Robert E. Alberti and Michael L. Emmons

Full Catastrophe Living: Using the Wisdom of Your Body and Mind to Face Stress, Pain, and Illness
Jon Kabat-Zinn, Ph.D.

The Healing Power of the Mind: Simple Exercises for Health, Well-Being, and Enlightenment
Tulku Thondup

Autobiography of a Yogi
Parmahansa Yogananda

Awake in the Dream
Lynne Miller

Bhagavad Gita: The Song of God
Swami Prabhavananda & Isherwood edition

A Buddhist Bible
Dwight Goddard

The Dhammapada
(Shambhala pocket edition)

The Diamond in Your Pocket
Gangaji

The Eternal Companion – Brahmananda
Swami Prabhavananda (Vedanta Press)

The Gospel of Sri Ramakrishna
"M", Ramakrishna (Vivekananda Center)

Graceful Exits: How Great Beings Die
Shushila Blackman

The Great Path of Awakening
Jamgon Kongtrul

The Hidden Messages in Water
Masaru Emoto and David A. Thayne

The Hobbit & The Lord of the Rings Trilogy
J.R.R. Tolkien

How to Win Friends and Influence People
Dale Carnegie

The I Ching
Wilhelm-Baynes translation

Lady of the Lotus-Born: The Life and Enlightenment of
Yeshe Tsogyal
Gyalwa Changchub & Namkhai Nyingpo

The Lives and Liberation of Princess Mandarava
Translated by Janet Gyatso

Shankara's Crest Jewel of Discrimination
*Translated by Swami Prabhavananda and
Christopher Isherwood*

Surfing the Himalayas
Dr. Frederick Lenz (Rama)

Snowboarding to Nirvana
Dr. Frederick Lenz (Rama)

The Tibetan Book of the Dead
W.Y. Evans-Wentz, Oxford Univ. Press

Tibetan Book of Living and Dying
Sogyal Rinpoche

Tibet's Great Yogi Milarepa
W.Y. Evans-Wentz

The Way of Life
Lao Tzu

A Way of Light
Kelly McTavish

The Upanishads: Breath of the Eternal
Translated by Swami Prabhavananda and
Frederick Manchester

Worlds of Power, Worlds of Light
Jenna Sundell

Zen Mind, Beginner's Mind
S. Suzuki

Musical Artists For Meditation

      Music is an excellent tool for meditation. The sound of the music can carry us through different mind states and feelings. It can also provide a blanket to protect us from the world while we open up during meditation. Music is also a wonderful timekeeper, so we can let go and not worry about how long we've been sitting.

      When selecting music for meditation, I use the smile test. I'll put a smile on my face, and then play the music. If I can hold my smile, then I'll use it for meditation. My tastes change from time to time, so if something doesn't work now, I'll try again a few months or years later. I also reserve my meditation music just for meditation.

Amethystium
David Arkenstone
Ian Anderson – *Divinities: Twelve Dances with God*
Jean Michael Jarre
Joaquin Lievano
Jonathan Goldman – *The Lost Chord*
Kitaro
Mozart
Patrick O'Hearn
Richard Buxton
Stephen Halpern
Tangerine Dream
Vivaldi
Vangelis
Zazen

Movies

Movies are a portal into different worlds, where we can experience many mind states and discover brand new ways of perceiving life. In the space of just a couple of hours, we can live an entire lifetime, and sometimes multiple lifetimes. Whether you watch alone or share the experience with others, movies are a treasure. When I need to rest, a great movie is the best gift. Here are some of my favorites that I could watch over and over.

12 Monkeys
After Earth
The Adjustment Bureau
Armageddon
A Beautiful Mind
Beyond Rangoon
Big
The Big Blue
Bruce Almighty
Chronicles of Riddick
Click
The Day After Tomorrow
Dogma
Dracula (Bram Stoker's)
E.T.
The Fifth Element
Finding Nemo
Forest Gump
Fried Green Tomatoes
Fun with Dick and Jane

Harry Potter *the books are great too!
The Hitchhikers Guide to the Galaxy
Inception
Interview with a Vampire
Joe vs. the Volcano
Jumanji
K-PAX
The Last Samurai
Lord of the Rings *trilogy*
Made In Heaven
The Matrix *trilogy*
Meet Joe Black
Meet the Robinsons
Memoirs of a Geisha
Men in Black *I & II & III*
Ocean's Eleven (+ Twelve + Thirteen)
Pirates of the Caribbean *trilogy*
Pitch Black
The Prestige
The Right Stuff
The Seventh Sign
Shrek
The Sixth Sense
Sky Captain and the World of Tomorrow
Spiderman *trilogy*
Starship Troopers
Star Trek – *all the old ones and the new ones*
Star Wars *trilogy (x2)*
Stigmata
Stranger Than Fiction
Terminator *trilogy*
Thelma and Louise

Titanic
Toys
Vanilla Sky
What the Bleep Do We Know!?
Wild, Wild West
Zathura: A Space Adventure

Websites

Whenever joining or using an Internet support group or website, or other newsgroup, you may want to first set up a separate email account (not the one you use on a regular basis), since you can open yourself to "spam" by posting on groups like this. Many sites, like www.Yahoo.com and www.Google.com offer free email accounts, which you can use to create your newsgroup account. Always protect your personal information such as your phone number, your street address, and any financial information.

Be careful about staying on the computer too long – remember to practice Pacing!

Author's Blog
www.jennasundell.com
Check out the Peace with Pain category for more articles about managing pain.

American Academy of Pain Management
www.aapainmanage.org

American Chronic Pain Association
www.theacpa.org   Phone: 1-800-533-3231
American Chronic Pain Association has great tools for logging, describing, and tracking pain to help you discuss your symptoms with your doctors. From the Home page go to → Pain Management Tools then → Communication Tools

American Fibromyalgia Syndrome Association
www.afsafund.org

American Pain Foundation
www.painfoundation.org

American Pain Society
www.ampainsoc.org

The Body Chronic
http://bodychronic.blogspot.com

Centers for Disease Control and Prevention
www.cdc.gov

CranioSacral Massage Information and Therapist Database
www.upledger.com
www.craniosacraltherapy.org

Facebook
www.facebook.com
Facebook can be used to connect with people you knew long ago, as well as to meet others with shared interests. Keep in mind anything you post anywhere on the Internet becomes public information and can be shared with anyone. Be sure to update your Privacy Settings within Facebook to your preferred level, and check them often as they can change when Facebook launches a new update. People post all sorts of weird, sometimes disturbing, interesting, and inspiring things. I do my best to share only inspiration; you can find me at facebook.com/jennasundellauthor

Feldenkrais Information and Classes
www.feldenkrais.com

Fibromyalgia Network
www.fmnetnews.com

Mayo Clinic Website
www.mayoclinic.com

Medicare
www.Medicare.gov

Meditation Instruction & Inspiration
www.dharmacenter.com
www.jennasundell.com
www.ramalila.com
www.ramalila.org
www.imeditate.com
www.zenmasterrama.com
www.meditationclub.com
www.americanbuddha.com
www.ramameditationsociety.org (free mp3 lectures!)
www.FrederickLenzFoundation.org
www.zazen.com
www.joaquinmusic.com/onemindmusic/music.html
www.bleepstore.com

National Cancer Institute
www.cancer.gov

National Chronic Pain Society
www.ncps-cpr.org

National Fibromyalgia Association
www.fmaware.org
www.fibrohope.org

National Women's Health Resource Center
www.womenshealth.gov

RX List - Prescription Medication Information
www.rxlist.com

Sleep Review: The Journal for Sleep Specialists
www.sleepreviewmag.com
(search for your medical condition)

Social Security Disability
www.ssa.gov/disability

The TMJ Association
www.tmj.org

U.S. National Library of Medicine
www.nlm.nih.gov/medlineplus

WebMD - General Medical Information and some discussion groups
www.webmd.com

Jenna Sundell

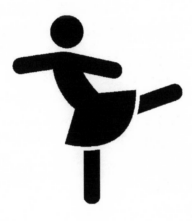

About The Author

Jenna Sundell, ordained as a monk of the Rama Lineage, began offering public meditation classes in 1994 after receiving a teaching empowerment. As her body started to fail due to a combination of chronic illnesses, she became disabled and could no longer work as a computer consultant. This experience allowed her to focus full time on her Buddhist practice, as well as teaching and writing. Jenna experiences constant pain, extreme ecstasy and profound peace, all at the same time each and every day.

In 1998, she co-founded Dharma Center, where she teaches Practical American Buddhism. While Dharma Center's main mission is to provide meditation and mindfulness training for people who live and work in the world, Jenna is also able to serve those who are physically suffering. Over the years, many students have thrived because they learned how to use meditation and mindfulness to manage their energy and their symptoms. In short, these students have learned to live as she does: unreasonably happy in a body overrun with pain.

Jenna's first book, *Worlds of Power, Worlds of Light* has inspired people from all walks of life to discover their spiritual path. Even years after its publication, people continue to encounter her first book and be motivated by it to begin their own spiritual search.

In an effort to share meditation with as many

people as possible, Jenna offers classes throughout the country. She also writes inspirational and educational posts on her blog, as well as on Facebook and Twitter.

Jenna's hobbies include writing poetry and exploring the mountains and deserts of Southern California by Jeep. She also practices Tai Chi and has fun with digital photography.

www.jennasundell.com
www.Facebook.com/jennasundell
www.Facebook.com/jennasundellauthor
www.twitter.com/jennasundell

Made in the USA
Middletown, DE
05 September 2019